To

Shirley and Ange

My Rocks

REVIEWS

My Year with Cancer by Robert Paul Quinn

I could not put it down. I didn't expect a book about cancer to make me laugh out loud, but it did. The humour lightened the mood while still telling the story. The author has managed to find the right balance between conveying their personal experience/opinions while remaining non-judgemental. The author is very open and honest and takes you on his personal journey to beat cancer. It provides an in-depth look at the good, bad and ugly side of cancer. There are some helpful and handy tips that some may find useful when trying to come to terms with fighting the disease. An excellent read with a dash of humour thrown in for good measure makes this an essential book for everyone who is either going through cancer treatment and/or friends/family who want to provide the right support for them.

David T

A very powerful account of one man's journey through the complex NHS system after being diagnosed with cancer. Never losing his sense of humour throughout, you will find this book both fascinating and insightful. The author is very relatable which kept me hooked right from the start.

Shirley Harvey

This book is a honest account of one man's journey from diagnosis and subsequent recovery from cancer. Don't be put off by the title, it's not all gloom and doom. I had thought it was going to be sad and serious but this is not the case. It's honest, funny and informative.

Mary Boyle

TABLE OF CONTENTS

Chapter One

Diagnosis – and the Dead Parrot Sketch!

I remember being wheeled into the recovery area of the endoscopic unit at QEQM hospital, in Margate, in a kind of 'where am I?' daze. Looking around, I noticed I was the only person in there, despite there being about ten bays. After ten minutes or so (I think), the doctor who carried out my procedure came to see me with a couple of nurses. At this point I should like to quote exactly what the doctor said, but, either owing to the effects of the sedative's wearing off or because of the impact of the sentence, I cannot exactly remember, but it was, 'We have found a malignant tumour on your oesophagus.' There was then some arm-rubbing (by them, not me); even I didn't feel prone to making any moves at that time! I was then left alone to absorb this information.

After about five minutes, a lady was wheeled into the room, placed in a bay and had the curtains pulled round her. Then another man was brought in and was put in a bay a couple down from me; a nurse was discussing something with him, but I couldn't quite focus on the context. The next thing I heard was the most almighty rumbling wet fart that I have heard in ages, coming from the lady's enclosed bay. This was one of those bottom-belches that any bloke on a Saturday afternoon down the pub with his friends would have been given supreme bragging-rights over. The fact that the nurses had enclosed the woman in curtains only added to the dramatic effect, as the curtains rippled like bed sheets on the washing line on a day with weather predicted by Michael Fish! I looked to my right to see the reaction to this event from the nurse and the other chap: I suppose looking for some light relief from my personal situation. However, it appeared as if I had imagined it. 'Hang on,' I thought, if I imagined that, perhaps I also imagined the conversation with the doctor ... Bloody sedative making me imagine things. I was just attempting to make my mind agree with this new set of information when the lady's curtains again fluttered like a plastic shopping-bag caught in a tree during a hurricane. This one was even louder, but still not a single reaction from the guy and the nurse, let alone an apology from the woman. 'I know what's going on,' I thought. 'I'm in a bloody Monty Python sketch.' I was just waiting for a load of blokes dressed in cardinal's cassocks to come in a chorus-line dancing, telling me that no-one expects the Spanish inquisition! The simple fact was that any kind of endoscopy/colonoscopy procedure has the unfortunate side-effect of making you fart, as I suddenly remembered from the pre-procedure literature and later discovered myself, once the sedative had fully worn off. The bloke in the next bay was either as shocked as myself but too embarrassed to react, as we blokes do by guffawing to each other, as the nurse was talking to him, or he himself was also receiving some not too pleasant news. I personally hope it was the first.

This sudden realisation brought me back to the little bay I was in and my own set of circumstances. Now I know the doctor said a malignant tumour, and I'm pretty bright, so I know that's not good at all, and the big C word is spinning in my head: but did she use it? Besides, surely there must be a test that gets done to ensure the diagnosis before that C word is used, isn't there? I've seen the dramas/films: you have a test or procedure, then go back to the docs two weeks later and leave their office either dancing around like a lucky git whose six numbers have come up, or with a face that looks like it's been slapped with a wet fish because a totally different set of numbers have given a totally different result. Either way, surely they couldn't know immediately, could they? Later on, I realised why it was a doctor doing the test and not a nurse. My GP had suspected cancer but obviously had not said anything to me until the endoscopy had been done and his suspicions were confirmed. The doctor who performed the procedure was, I believe, a specialist in this area and knew exactly what she was looking at, so there really wasn't much doubt. I had spoken to her briefly prior to the endoscopy, and she had been talking about the fact that the referral was a partial one and she would like to do some blood-tests and possibly a colonoscopy as well.

'What are you going to do?' I asked. 'Spin the table round after the first check?!' Back in my Monty Python sketch, a nurse came to speak to me to check how the information was sinking in, and I tentatively asked the big question that hadn't been directly answered up until now.

'So is it cancer, then?'

'Yes, I'm afraid,' she replied.

'Bugger,' I thought.

Chapter Two

About Me

My name is Robert Paul Quinn, but the Robert was a kind of family heirloom, and as both my father and I used to crap ourselves when my mother screamed 'Robert!', I soon became Paul to avoid any confusion over blame. This simple fact was to become quite a bugbear of mine during the present period of my life: as anyone knows, the 'computer' has your full correct name, so all letters and bookings are made thus. Therefore all nurses/doctors/receptionists will call you by your first 'correct' name, as obviously 'the computer is never wrong'! Now if my treatment had been confined to one hospital, the request from me to be called Paul would eventually have been accepted, and I should not have heard myself constantly having to repeat the it's-a-family-heirloom-thing many, many times. Unfortunately, my treatment was destined to be spread across many different hospitals, dealt with by many staff, and I ended up giving in to the fact that, despite my asking, I was going to be called Robert, and, with a slight wince every time it was said, I accepted this.

I was born in sunny Paisley in September 1965, the first child of Robert Francis Quinn and Agnes Harvey Quinn. My father was a professional musician, and my mother was a mum. When I was about a year old, my father left the music scene of Glasgow and headed south, which brought him to the Beacholme holiday camp in Cleethorpes, where he spent the next twenty-odd years as leader of the resident band. We settled in; we had an addition: my sister, Shirley Anne Quinn; and that was us. I was quite a bright kid, but with no real ambition or focus (my parents, teachers and probably many friends would call me 'lazy-minded'!). I settled into my obvious role of class clown and chief pain to all around me. Being the child of someone working on the holiday-camp afforded me lots of access and privileges which I abused with aplomb. The years went by, and I scraped through, and at the age of seventeen I joined the RAF as a policeman - which was a bad move, but hindsight is such an overrated thing. In any case, it fitted in to the great scheme of stumbling from one bad decision to another! I left the RAF some five years later and returned home, to find my father now working in Spain, with my mother and Shirley there with him. This would have been perfect, me living in the family home alone, if I had had the resources to run a three-bedroomed bungalow on the little money I left the RAF with. Well, I bimbled on and over the years travelled much of this fine country, procuring various forms of employment, from kitchen salesman to sanitary-towel-machine-operator and eventually found myself some twenty-five-odd years ago (not sure whether I mean odd as in approximately, or as in just bloody odd times) living and working in the lovely coastal town of Dover. After many years of what some would call extreme fun and hedonistic behaviour, I found myself settled in a good job with a fantastic set of friends and a nice little flat overlooking the harbour. I have never really been in a proper relationship or had children. Never got round to truly settling down and growing up until ... maybe tomorrow! When everything is taken in context, I was quite lucky, considering the aimless way I had drifted for the previous many years. I smoked, I drank, and I occasionally dabbled in substances of dubious legal standing. I never really focused on the future, or indeed sometimes the present. Because I just thought I would shuffle off this mortal coil, and as I had no responsibility to children or a wife, that would be fine, and I didn't have to consider any financial or moral responsibilities. Well, that's the life synopsis. I should add that I have a very quick wit; a good sense of humour and a very caring and passionate side that I usually disguise in layers of sarcasm. I have a great singing voice; a natural ability for music, which I inherited from my father, and a psyche that continually reminds me of past errors and ensures I never forget or let go of these things. I have a close relationship with my God and strong moral beliefs which I try to live by, but mostly fail miserably at. 'The road to hell is paved with good intentions' should be put on my tombstone. Weird thing is, in these past months, it very nearly was!

The reason for a brief synopsis about me is that, for the purposes of this book, who I am is irrelevant. What I am trying to achieve here is to put down the events of my journey with cancer from diagnosis to present in the hope of helping myself move on, and in the great hope that others may be comforted and humoured and may understand aspects of such a journey a little better, enabling them to use the information to deal with their individual pathway a little more easily. I am not medically trained (although I am the office first-aider!) and will not advise that any medical decision is based on my experience. This is my journey: use it if you can to make your own a little more bearable.

Chapter Three
Initial Thoughts

Back in the recovery bays, the realisation that I had cancer was still spinning round my head like an irritating fly that I was sure I could swat away as soon as I got the sedatives out of my system. Eventually I shaped myself up, got dressed and started to leave the ward. Reality came back in the form of anxious looks from the nurses and their saying, rather hurriedly, that I could not leave just yet, as the doctor wanted to see me and I should wait in a side-room until called. I was also handed a form to fill in, to give feedback on my experience that day in the endoscopic unit. Damn: I'm back in the Python sketch. So I sat in the waiting-room ticking boxes … how did I rate the care I was given … was I furnished with enough information … would I recommend the disease to a friend (what a joke!)? All of a sudden I look up, and lo and behold, Mrs Windy Bottom wanders in, plonks herself down and says, 'Well, that wasn't very nice, was it?' Suffice to say I buried myself in a detailed reply to How did I rate my experience, from 1 to Gale force 10?

I had come to the unit under the following circumstances, which I feel are an important part of this, because, as with everything, an early diagnosis is quite literally the difference between life and death. I had been having some difficulty with chest pains for a few weeks but had simply put it down to the fact that my sister was getting married in the May of 2013, and I was stressing myself a little too much about trying to be the perfect big brother on her great day. Both our parents had by now unfortunately passed away, and it had taken me and my sister a while to reconnect with each other, so I put a little too much pressure on myself. The wedding took place, and we had a fantastic time. My sister looked beautiful, and the whole event was incredible; including the pre-wedding Scottish and Cleethorpes contingents coming together in a truly breath-taking show of solidarity in partying. I know it sounds silly, but I somehow knew the pain I was experiencing wasn't to do with my heart, but, when it continued post-wedding, I decided I had better have a chat with my GP.

The first visit confirmed my suspicions, and I was diagnosed with digestive problems, specifically indigestion. This is something I had never experienced previously, apart from after a twelve-hour session - and I don't mean down the gym. So off I went with my prescription pills and thought no more of it. The next few weeks I got on with things. I was feeling good about myself as I had started to lose a few pounds. Pinch an inch? I could yank a yard. My office had recently moved, and I didn't see the point in buying a car for a couple of miles' journey each way, so I put my moral-crusading best green bonnet on and joined a 'bike to work' scheme. I was really enjoying it, apart from the odd bum-hole car/van driver (I'm sure they would say the same about me), and I put the weight loss down to the twenty-five or so miles I was doing each week. The problem was that the pain was not easing, and my appetite was not great; despite my sixteen-stone frame, I wasn't the biggest eater. The biggest issue, though, was that every time I saw someone, especially after getting off my bike (bugger off, Tebbit: I'm not getting back on it - slight political gag for readers of my generation!), they always commented on how pale I looked. Well, after a few times of being compared to a cast-off corpse on a film about a vampiric rampage, I thought I had better get back to the doc's. This time I had some blood drawn and waited to find out whether indigestion really could turn you into an albino. The very next day I got a call at work and headed back to my GP to discover that I was anaemic. 'Bugger,' I thought, 'how the hell did I get myself pregnant?' My doctor then tapped his pencil and explained to me that this was a symptom rather than a cause; that there was obviously a small bleed somewhere internally, and he was going to refer me for an endoscopy to see what the problem was. 'Excellent,' I thought, 'at least we're getting there.' My thinking was a small ulcer, leaking like a tap that needed a new washer. The doctor's thoughts, as I later discovered when I was copied in on the letter to him giving the results of the endoscopy, was that 1+1=2. Weight loss plus discomfort plus internal bleeding (yes I know that's technically 1+1+1) = suspected cancer. Turned out he was right and I was wrong. Double bugger.

Eventually I was called by the nurse, but not to go in and see the doctor just yet. They wanted to know who had come over with me, as they wished to have a word with them. This person was Angela Knight, a girl whom I had known for all my time in Dover, and I shall mention her quite frequently during this book, as she proved to be more than just a good friend throughout the coming months. Ange went out of her way to take me to many appointments and also to listen to me when things got a bit much, but, more importantly, she helped me keep a sense of perspective about it all and supported me greatly when things were not going so well: a great friend, and also the ex-partner of one of my other friends. Trust me, the interrelationships involved in good friendships can be quite staggering, not to mention awkward, but, when we are as awesome as I am, we get round these things. OK, friends make allowances for us. Now, as I say, Ange is a great friend, but she is not my partner, so I point this out to the nurse. By this time the doctor has returned and tells me that they would prefer to talk to Ange regardless of our relationship, and I could come into the room or not - this being said as the door was slowly, caringly but firmly closed on me! I stood in the corridor with a million thoughts running through my head. I had always thought (and please don't kid yourself: we all have thoughts of how we should deal with cancer if it ever popped its ugly head into our lives) that I should tell no-one. Simple. I should deal with it the best I could, and I should carry on with my life as if nothing had happened. Quite how I should explain the symptoms and treatment I hadn't quite thought through, but as Baldrick would say, 'I have a cunning plan.' My plan, however, was denial. No, not a holiday to Egypt, but the total bury-my-head-in-the-sand ostrich plan.

So there I was, stood in a corridor, having my plan dissolved in the first few moments of diagnosis, without so much as any proper input into the situation. A few moments later, the door opened, and I was invited in. 'Sure I'm not intruding?' were the words on my lips, but the sight of Ange stopped me in my tracks. Being a very strong person who just gets on with things ('yes, yes,' I hear the women shout, 'that's what we do,') it was quite the reality-check to see her looking as weepy as someone who has just watched a 1940 black-and-white film where the main character has just sacrificed themselves in the kind of noble way that modern films with their 'FX' just can't do. She came over, gave me a hug, and we both sat down with the nurse and the department sister. We confirmed the diagnosis, and I was given some literature; offered the chance to ask questions and advised of what should happen in the immediate future as to my treatment. They had taken some biopsies, and I should be advised of the results later. We then left the department. Again I got an arm-rub off the ward-sister, only this time I noticed she was very attractive, although by now I didn't really care, as I felt like the sad balloons you see flapping around funfairs with only a fraction of the air left in them.

Ange took me home and came in for a cuppa. There were a lot of held-back tears and slips into grown-up this-is-what-we'll-do mode, but it was mainly a sense of shock filling the flat. After making sure I would be OK and promising to come back later after work, Ange left, and, for the first time since childhood, I now lived in my flat with another. Unfortunately, the other was cancer, and a quick eviction wasn't on the cards. I must have sat for a while just blankly looking out at the sea, letting the day lap over me like the waves. I then thought: 'OK, time to let some people know.' Again, my big plan had been blasted away, probably by the woman in the Monty Python sketch! Keep your humour people; by gum, you're going to need it. It was as I picked up the phone to call my sister that I looked at it, put it down and then scratched my head thinking, Did they *really* say cancer? Did I mishear? Did they say they thought it might be? I went from being organised in my head, knowing whom I was going to tell, why and what, to doubting that I was even ill in the first place. I felt like the contestants on *Millionaire* who know the answer but just can't seem to get the words past their lips in case they are wrong and because there's just too much at stake. This, however, wasn't for £32,000: this was a real life-changer, so I had to be sure before I put it out there. I texted Ange, and the reply came back, 'Yes, hun, sorry.' It was then that I realised why they had taken her into the room and told her what was happening. Quite simply, on your own, you cannot process the information straightaway. Self-preservation will create doubt and confusion to the point you will even begin to wonder if the events had occurred and ask yourself why you had a phone in your hand. The reason I struggled so much with making the calls was quite simply that I was terrified: not of the cancer itself, as I had no idea as yet of the extent or prognosis, but I was terrified of putting that word 'out there'. If I was wrong, or there had been a mistake, which can happen (I thought hopefully), then it is a lot harder to put things back into Pandora's box than it is to let them out. After confirmation from Ange, though, I knew that it was real. It was happening, and, worst of all, it was cancer. The way I tried to tell my sister, other family and friends was in a positive way: 'It's early days, treatments have come a long way, I'm sure it's all going to be fine ... ' but the truth is, I just didn't know. I think I told about six people and then work. Each time, as I rolled the words over in my head, the day seemed to click together like seeing the pieces of a puzzle fall into place. Acceptance allowed itself into my brain, and I began formulating a plan. As I said, I'm not a doctor, but the seed of a plan nurtured itself into me, and I could at least see a way through the next phase.

The next morning I woke, and it was a bit surreal, as there were certain things I thought would happen but didn't. In my head I thought I should wake groggy from the previous day's events, but I didn't. My mind was quite clear; I have cancer. I thought I should have one of those eureka moments where I should hear more clearly the birds singing, or the sea crashing. I thought I should crystallise everything in my mind, and serenity would calm me, but the simple truth is, it didn't happen. I simply woke on Friday the 26th July 2013 knowing that I had a malignant tumour on my oesophagus. I wasn't in a Hollywood weepy: this was my life, and this was the reality. As I will say throughout this book, this is how I felt, and this is what I experienced. There will be common ground; otherwise I should not be sharing this. Hopefully that common ground will help or even prepare you, but I believe there are about 200 types of cancer, and I very much doubt whether each cancer reacts or works on individuals in the same way each time. There is no right or wrong, to my mind, in how we deal with it, as long as we do deal with it.

Well, the next day was a pretty strange one, to be honest. I had the day of convincing myself it was really happening and I had told the truth to those I needed to. I still hadn't put it into the wider public domain, as I wanted to know all the facts and have a better understanding of the bigger picture before I did that. This was in no way a slur on friends whom I hadn't told. It was a simple plan in my mind. Get all the information I can at this stage. Tell it to the people I had already informed of my diagnosis and ask them to pass it along. Friends tell friends, family tell family, and soon enough people know and you haven't had to have the conversation a hundred times. I don't say this to be flippant; it is just that telling people is very, very difficult, no matter how you do it. I found it extremely upsetting, because I felt that I was putting a huge burden on to them. I was not being a martyr in any way, shape or form, but I felt responsible. That may seem like a strange thing to say, or maybe it's not. I don't know. All I can do is let you know how it affected me. These are important people to me, and I cared deeply about them and how this would affect them. It felt as if I was making myself vulnerable as well and seeming weak. The point is that we will all have these feelings and others, but it will depend on the individual and the circumstance. The important thing is that the feelings are true for you.

The next thing that happened was that I felt a huge sense of acceptance: not of the disease but of my own mortality and the practicalities of death. Who would arrange my funeral? Would I get cremated? How will people cope? (Bit selfish but, hey, I like to think I'm popular!) But more importantly, who would pay? This was an important consideration to me, because my sister and I had lost both parents, and we were well aware of the expense involved in a funeral. I knew one thing, and that was that my sister would not have to suffer the financial burden of paying for mine. I am covered for a fair amount if I die whilst employed by the company I work for, but, just to be sure, I contemplated getting as much as possible from payday lenders and using it for costs. After all, those old buggers in the loan adverts should go before me, right? I wonder what the APR is on eternity.

Obviously I would not have done that and I don't condone it in any way, but the thought did cross my mind. I think that, in my case anyway, once you take on board the initial information that you have cancer, the brain needs to organise and make sense of this new set of data. I found myself trying to shuffle it in my head so that it made a little more sense and I could therefore move forward, knowing I was as prepared as I could be for the next stage of things, no matter how dark or light they may be. What did help me enormously, in the strangest way, was planning the actual service myself. I had the programme in my mind. 'In my life' by the Beatles as people arrive. Then there would be a speech. I thought about this and decided that the best thing was not to put someone through the trauma of having to say out loud how completely awesome I was: I should take the opportunity to do it myself! I chuckled as I pictured my family and friends sitting there listening to the priest and then … out would come my voice. I made it light and funny so as to take away a little of the seriousness of the moment for people. I thanked them all and tried to encourage them to use my situation in any way they could in their own lives, to make things a little better: the usual noble sort of thing, so you hope you are remembered, even in some small way. After the speech, my next song would be 'Always look on the bright side of life' by, yes, you guessed it, Monty Python! I was, and still am, unsure of the last song, but I'm leaning to either 'My Way,' Sinatra, or 'Fix You' by Coldplay. People would then go back somewhere, have some nibbles, drink copious amounts of alcohol and hopefully have fun and wax lyrical about times with me. I haven't exactly made a huge impact on this wonderful planet we have (earlier reference to being lazy-minded) but I should like to think that I have made a small difference to the people I have met. As I said at my father's funeral, 'If at some point in the future you should think of me with a smile on your face, then I'll be happy wherever I am.'

Well, that was the funeral sorted, and next I sorted in my mind that I would put into letters my thoughts to some close people. This is something that I should recommend to all. I don't know whether it is the British reserve or whether it's just me that's crap at communicating effectively when it really matters, but, whatever your belief, religion, creed, colour, political leaning, wealth or sexual orientation, I believe that the most important thing we should all remember is that the only thing that matters is each other. I don't mean that in a let's-all-link-arms-and-sing-Kum-ba-Ya sort of happy-clappy way. One thing I truly believe is that People in the singular are absolutely brilliant. Obviously there are exceptions, like Simon Cowell, but individual human beings are mostly fantastic. People in the plural sense are … well, crap. We find reason to fight, argue and pretty much make our own lives pretty poo. This is something I found to be quite accurate in my dealings with the NHS, but more on that later. So getting across to certain people in your life, on an individual basis, just how important they are to you is, I believe, very helpful. It doesn't have to be long and soppy, it just has to be from the heart and meant. It will help you, and it will undoubtedly help them. Still, you could always break the mould and tell them face to face prior to any permanent separation! No thanks, not enough Bacardi in the world for that. So that was me. Day one was acceptance of what I had found out, and day two was a pretty strange way of trying to make sense of it and organise myself. The next thing I had to do was get the medical wheels rolling, but, as with a lot of my treatment over the coming months, this was not going to be easy.

Chapter Four

The Plan

The diagnosis was made on the Thursday, and the next important step was for me to have a CT scan. The purpose of this was to see the initial spread of the cancer, if any. The scan was duly booked for the Saturday, and the next step would be for my case to be brought before a multi-discipline team-meeting, which for medical cases was held on a Monday. These meetings are a coming-together of specialist nurses/oncology specialists/surgical teams etc., and probably in the corner there will be a machine that goes 'bing'. (Sorry, can't seem to stray from the Monty Python themes at present!) There is also a surgical multi-disciplinary meeting, and that apparently is held on a Wednesday. I went to the QEQM hospital on the Saturday with Ange and was duly directed to a lovely NHS dressing-gown and a chair outside the CT room. I don't know about you, but things like CT scan/ECG/CAT scan etc. were terms I was familiar with but still sounded a bit *Star Wars*-ish and a little scary. The CT scanner is a big vertical doughnut-shaped device that whirs around the area to be checked, making you feel as if you are the filling in some strange medical experiment to make a real RoboCop-type cyborg. Before you go into the scanner, you get injected with a liquid (I'm not 100% sure what that is), but it allows them to see what the medical team are looking for a lot more clearly. During a lot of these sorts of tests and procedures, they will inject or get you to drink various things to help with the tests. Personally, I should have been more than happy to fill up regularly with liquid, but I don't think Bacardi shows up quite so clearly. The liquid they injected on this occasion apparently has a different reaction for males and females; apparently it makes girls feel as if they need to pee. With me it was like taking a large glass of something nice and strong on a cold day. You know that warm feeling that seeps into you? However, I did have an entirely different feeling during a CT scan much later on in my treatment. That one made me feel as if I had had a trouser accident. I was that convinced that I had made no.2 on the trolley you lie on that I hesitated and made sure the nurse had turned away before having a discreet look underneath me to make sure the department didn't have to be closed for some severe industrial cleaning. Fortunately it was just a sensation, and the trolley was indeed minus any traces of my bodily functions, so, with a silly sense of relief, I confessed my worry to the nurse, dressed as quickly as I could and bolted for the door more quickly than a lottery winner on his way to cash the cheque and tell his bank manager how he really feels about him.

Well, that was the scan done, so all I had to do now was wait for my appointment with the specialist nurse who would advise me of the results of both the discussion in the multi-discipline meeting and my CT scan. I had been told in the chat after diagnosis that the specialist nurse would ring me on the Monday afternoon after the meeting; which in my case would be a week Monday after the CT scan. The reality was (and it made total sense with hindsight) that the case would not be discussed on the Monday over the phone, but an appointment would be made for the Tuesday afternoon.

As I mentioned earlier, I expected there to be some dramatic test initially and then a two week wait for the doctor to look at you all doe-eyed, like Bambi, whilst lowering their voice and passing you the C card. For me that didn't happen, as I have explained. The reality is, though, that there will be several periods over the course of treatment where you do have to suffer these agonising waits. This ten-day period between the CT scan and my meeting with the specialist nurse was to be the first of many for me. I think it's important that you prepare for these periods, as they can be very self-destructive, and, if not handled in the right way, they can drastically add to the stress and suffering of it all for yourself and those around you. The first thing to remember is that, although you are classed as a priority within the NHS, I believe the Service work to a two-week rule for most of these types of things. For a body as complex and intricate as the NHS, that is great, but to an individual who has had their world distorted beyond imagination, every second now not only seems vitally important but also changes from lasting what seems like an hour to a millisecond dependent on the circumstance; and it can seem an age. The thing I tried through my experience of these types of situations, albeit not very successfully, was not to overreact. It's easy to get lost in the time and focus on the negatives. Now that may lead you to doing something as simple as smashing down the garden-shed that you've wanted to do for ages but were always unsure about, to going on rampant alcohol binges (thank you for getting me through that period, Mr Dyer, lol). From thinking it's all doom and gloom and what the hell, who really cares anyway? to dumping your spouse and buying a sports car, which you then wrap round a tree, having combined this with the previous point and therefore saved the NHS thousands on your treatment.

The important thing to bear in mind here is that we are all very different people: 'one man's meat' etc., and the circumstances you find yourself in, if you should ever be unlucky enough to have to face this disease, can vary drastically. Some victims are surrounded by wealth and loving families, whereas some may find themselves in a bedsit with a phone that never bleeps and a real sense of isolation, or you may be somewhere in the middle, like myself. What I learned from these periods was to try not to focus too much on the worst-case scenario. This may seem an obvious thing to say, but it really is a pretty difficult thing to do. Since cancer doesn't care about the individual, take this time and use it to consider one very important fact: do you want to beat it? I know there will be a lot of people that will think this is a totally stupid question, because of course they wish to beat it, but trust me, it is not quite that simple. As I stated previously, there are many different types of cancer, and unfortunately not everyone survives. This is dependent on many factors, and unfortunately a lot of people do not get to ask themselves this question, which makes your answer even more pertinent. Throughout this book I have resigned myself to the fact that if I am going to make it useful to both myself and the reader, I am going to have to be very truthful. I don't mean in the good ol' American way of having a discussion about everything that happens.

'I just bought some Tampax at the drug store.' 'Yeah, but how do you feeeeel about it?'

I mean that sometimes we think or experience things in our lives that we know are not normal. They go against the grain of what we perceive to be us as individuals, but nevertheless they exist and are real. One such thing is our own mortality. I think most of us (if not, I really hope you are a very small minority) would consider it in our hearts a truly admirable thing if we could choose exactly how we were to cash in our chips. To push a child away from disaster and sacrifice ourselves at the same time would be a justifiable end, would it not? This is not about religious martyrdom or anything similar: it is just that I believe that, when it comes down to it, if we had a choice, we should all like to think that we could be that person. The unfortunate fact with cancer is that sometimes you do have that choice. It's not that I wanted to roll over and slip away, or that my life was so awful that I saw an easy way out: it's quite simply that when I looked my own mortality in the face, I found myself asking these questions: was this meant to be? do I really have the fight in me? can I really use this as an excuse just to give up? The fact that I am now writing this book will let you know how I answered. How will you?

The Sunday before my appointment with the specialist nurse, a couple of my friends decided it would be therapeutic for me to accompany them for some lunch along the seafront and see how the day went. So I took a stroll across the road at lunchtime to meet my friends Lee and Mof. One of the major issues I was having at that time was my difficulty in swallowing food. Certain things were fine, but things like bread (toast was fine, strangely enough) or meats like steak and pork chops would leave me in absolute agony. This makes sense, really, as. if you have a large tumour in your gullet, things have to squeeze past. It's a bit like the skinny bloke trying to get on stage past the relatives in any episode of Jeremy Kyle. Another reason I was quite lucky was that my tumour was positioned towards the bottom of my gullet, so the food could pass by it into the opening of my stomach. Some people have theirs nearer the neck, and I can only imagine the problems they encounter. It was even discussed with me that a stent (I believe a surgical bypass of an obstruction) or even a tube (a replacement entirely) could be put in place, but fortunately it never came to that.

So I was a little dubious about a meal, but again this is where I have to be honest. The real intention that day was not to be sociable in any way. I knew this was going to be a session. They knew this was going to be a session, but you have to do the dance to make it to the table. I think I settled for a toasted bacon sandwich, of which I ate about half, but the pee-taking really started when I ordered a glass of Pinot. I tried to make out it was because it was a lovely sunny Sunday sitting on the seafront, and that's what I fancied. The truth is there was absolutely no way I could physically swallow beer, as gassy things were also on my no-no list. We did the usual thing blokes do in these situations and took the mick out of each other, and eventually it was decided we should go to a friend's pub the other side of town where we knew we could be loud and boys, and not upset anyone, apart from Lee's bank manager! I was quite apprehensive about this, because, as I said, there were only certain people that knew about my 'condition', Lee and Mof being two. I do know a lot of people who drink in the pub we were going to, so my concern was that I should get a little too drunk and blab to the world.

Anyway, we headed to the pub, and all was well with the world; they even managed to find a half-decent bottle of white. Pity they didn't have a single wine-glass! Later on, as we moved (no, not pubs, from wine to Bacardi), I began to sense that some people knew more than I thought, and I was pretty sure it hadn't been me with the loose lips. It turned out that one of my other friends, Chris, who was not with us that day, had in fact been about as able to keep the news about me to himself as Billy the Supergrass is on Grassing Day in the month of Grasstober. By that time, however, the Bacardis were flowing, and the juke-box was blaring, and the reality was that I was getting my results in two days' time. So sod it: let's have a blow out; it may all go Pete Tong at the meeting. It was absolutely brilliant being with friends and doing what we normally do. No, Dr/Professor, not that many units in one week! It was only when the 'bucket list' was mentioned that I remembered what was happening to me. 'Drive an Aston Martin DB9 Volante and sing a couple of numbers with Jools Holland's big band' was my instant reply. I didn't need to have cancer to know how much I would love to do those things.

The next thing, however, is a little near the knuckle, but it is something that made me howl with laughter, though some may find it inappropriate. It depends on the friends you have, who you are and what makes you laugh, but, with us, this just about sums things up. I noticed a bit of paper floating around and assumed (I hate that word: 'ass out of you and me.' Mother of all cock-ups: I should have just used a different word, but I wanted to say how much I hate it!) that it was for football or darts or anything like that. How wrong I was! It was a sweepstake to guess the day I should take the Big Mortal Leap! What got me more than anything was that the bastards had picked all the good days, like Christmas Eve or New Year's Day. But the one that made me chuckle the most was the barman, who put simply '6.30 today'. Sorry, guys, still here, you all lost.

Well, the appointed Tuesday came, and I met Sue, a specialist oncology nurse at the Viking Day Unit at the QEQM hospital in Margate; not quite the Jolly Boys' outing I had wished for! Sue is the type of nurse you hope and pray exists in the NHS and quite frankly proved to be a bigger rock to me in the coming months then I could have imagined, but more on that later. The Viking Day Unit is one of those places that takes you by surprise the first time you see it. My first indication was not being able to find it in the main hospital building. It is a separate annex in the grounds. I'm not sure whether it is there for diplomatic protection of the patients who use it or for the patients who frequent the main hospital. Either way, when you sit in the reception-area and see your first lady wearing a head scarf, exactly where you are is brought home with a big bang. We went into Sue's office, and formalities were followed, and a file was created on me, which started out the size of a Jehovah's Witnesses' list of people who would invite them in for coffee and some months later would resemble an MP's expenses' form. Basics over, it was then explained to me that the news was that the CT scan and biopsies had shown early indications that the cancer was confined to my oesophagus and a few nodes in my stomach and had not spread further. My lungs and other organs appeared clear. It was at this point I had to apologise to Sue: how was I to know I should let out such a gust of air with my sigh of relief?

We then discussed the outcome of the multi-disciplinary meeting and therefore my course of treatment. What they wanted me to do was to agree to a set of procedures which I shall explain in more detail as they occur: a PET scan, a laparoscopy and an endoscopic ultrasound. And the unfortunate thing, as far as I was concerned, was that these strange things I had to undergo were not *treatments*. They were all tests of varying degrees of intrusiveness to determine the exact extent of my cancer and how best to treat it. She then explained that the ultimate aim was to establish its size, contain and shrink it with chemotherapy and then to have an operation to remove the tumour. We then discussed other things such as how I was feeling physically and how I was getting on generally with eating and work etc.

It's at this point that you realise you have to accept the course that will follow. You are effectively putting your life into their hands. I have always been extremely glad that we have an NHS and felt confident in them. I knew that any future I had lay with them, so I just accepted the plan I was given and hoped that it would all end in a positive way. The basic sense of the chat was there were two routes my treatment would take. I would be poked and prodded and hopefully the tumour would be contained. It would respond to chemotherapy and therefore become operable. The other route was not one I relished in any way. If it had spread more than initially thought or did not respond to the chemotherapy, treatment would be palliative. This word is not one I was overly familiar with prior to that moment, but I got the impression it was a polite way of dressing up some bad news: almost like putting a ball-gown on a sheep and taking the animal to the dance - you know it's still a sheep, no matter how many times she re-applies her lipstick. Palliative means that you will be treated with chemotherapy or radiotherapy and drugs etc. until they no longer work and then offered pain-relief. To me it means they will deal with the symptoms, but they cannot get rid of the cause. That could mean days, weeks or years dependent on the aggressiveness of the cancer and the type you have. I believe some people live many years undergoing palliative treatment, but for me I really hoped that was not a road I should have to walk. Like Sir Cliff, I didn't want to spend the rest of my life under the shadows. All the procedures and checks are eventually leading to a better understanding of your individual disease so that it can be 'staged' (given a numeric grading of the size and growth of the cancer) and treated in whatever way it can be. I left the meeting feeling a little numb, trying not to make eye-contact with the headscarf ladies, and we sat in Ange's car and mulled over the meeting. I was obviously as happy as a grease monkey on the all-women's international beach hockey team, because the cancer had not spread so far. However, it was now that I began to realise the intensity of the road ahead; but, hey-ho, at least there was a road.

Chapter Five

Starting the Procedures

The dates for the three procedures came in very quickly, considering. I received the letters giving details, and all were to happen over the next month or so. At first, I got the dates and was quite dismayed: 'Don't they know I've got cancer? I can't wait all this time just to see whether it's treatable.' One of the main frustrations I had during this period was timelines. As an individual you don't care if there are lots of patients all needing the NHS and its services: all you care about is yourself. The fact is that the care-plan you are given is usually pretty considerate of your individual circumstances, and you have to accept it and try to cope in your own way with whatever demons pop up from time to time. However, there are times when things can drift, and a proactive stance is definitely a requirement, but that is down to individual circumstance, and I shall discuss that later.

First Procedure

Well, the first procedure on my list was a PET scan (Positron Emission Tomography), which is a machine similar to the CAT scanner, but this time, instead of a dye of types, you are injected with a radioactive liquid. I believe this is because it locks on to the cancerous cells in the body like a vapid woman to a sixty-year-old guy driving a Ferrari. (I cast no aspersions on either vapid women or Ferraris.) If you buy enough copies of this, then I hope to have both! As with all of these procedures and appointments, since the medical team will always want to see lists of any medication you are taking, I found it very handy to type it into my phone and just add items as they were prescribed. One more silly thing is, always take the letter for the appointment with you when you attend. We are talking about the NHS here. I always thought bureaucracy was a small fishing village in Cornwall until I encountered the full might of the NHS.

My PET scan was to be done at Canterbury Hospital. You are advised that you will be given the injection and will have to sit still for about an hour before the scan is done. You are also advised that you cannot be in contact with pregnant women or small children for approximately four hours post-procedure. My scan was done in a converted lorry-trailer at the back of the hospital. A few questions were asked, and some checks were done, which included a blood-sugar test, as I am a type 2 diabetic. Now the thing is that I have not had many issues with my diabetes: it is pretty well under control, but, as I stated previously, I was diagnosed because I was anaemic, and my levels had become really low the previous week, so my GP had requested I have a blood transfusion. This was done at the QEQM Hospital, Margate, over a period of eighteen hours, and this itself should have given me a glimpse into the occasionally strange workings of the NHS. I had an appointment to meet my oncologist as well that day, so went to the hospital early, thinking they would hook me up with a few pints of the red stuff and that would be fine. Unfortunately the time dragged by, and it was late afternoon by the time they got the first bag up; I was to receive three units in total. One thing that did confuse me, though, was that they were dripping blood slowly into me: I always thought that they put good blood in and pumped out the old rubbish. Apparently not, as they were topping me up to the correct level. Well, at least I gave the nurse a chuckle when I asked. Because of the lateness of the day, it was decided that I should be kept in, as they could not give me any blood overnight for safety reasons, and there was no way it would be finished that day.

So after being moved from the CDU (Clinical Decisions Unit), where they had started the transfusion, I was moved to a side ward in A&E, where I was now very happy, as it had a TV. Unfortunately bed shuffling is something we have all heard about, and, as they wanted to free up the ward for possible overnight extras from a dramatic episode of *Holby*, I was moved to a ward with no TV, just me and four poor souls with stark walls to stare at. I later realised that it was the stroke ward, but I never got touched up. I must say that, throughout my treatment, there have been a couple of individuals who take a few minutes to go out of their way to make things a little easier. One such person, and I don't even know her name, was the ward-sister the next day. After I had been sitting there bored as anything, it was about 2pm when the last drop of blood had been forced into my veins, but unfortunately they then had to send a sample to pathology to make sure it was all OK. This would have meant another four hours or so sitting in that ward. The kind ward-sister must have seen my notes and realised I was going to be seeing enough of hospitals over the next few months, so she said that, if I went to my GP the next day for a blood sample to be taken, she would be happy to let me go. I know she didn't do it for bed-shuffling: she did it for the reason that the vast majority of nurses and doctors work in the NHS - they really do care, but they just don't often get a chance to show it.

Anyway, I had to let you know about the transfusion, because, back at the PET scan lorry (sounds like something a well-known band from the 80s used to audition backing singers), the nurse was now testing my blood-sugar and, as she looked me sweetly in the eye with a big warm smile and said 'Well, Mr Quinn, that's a good one, 5.5,' I didn't have the heart to tell her that technically it wasn't my blood!

I then went into the corridor to be injected with my radioactive dye. Would I become invisible? Would I become super-strong, and would my farts melt steel? All these things were going through my mind as a nurse came towards me, not only carrying a lead-lined box but also extracting from it a lead-lined injector. As she injected me with the substance, I asked her, 'When will I get my superpowers, and will I get a comic straight away?' Now here is the flipside to some nurses: no sense of humour. Saying that, she had probably heard the same comment a dozen times previously, but for me, well, humour is my armour.

An hour or so later, I was put on to the trolley to be loaded into the scanner. I still hadn't started to glow green so was slightly deflated. That was probably a good thing, as it would make fitting me in a lot easier! The difference with this scan compared with the CT scan is that this one lasts about twenty minutes. Now that doesn't sound a long time as a giant doughnut whirrs round you in 5cm stages every few minutes, but trust me, as soon as you raise your arms above your head and are conveyed into the machine like some kind of alternative adrenalin ride at Chessington World of Adventures, you will find that immediately your nose starts to itch, your trousers need pulling up and an overwhelming urge to just bolt from it hits you; and I'm not claustrophobic. Well, it was soon over, so I took Ange to Waitrose for a quick bite to eat. Ange would not take any petrol-money, as usual, but settled for lunch and my paying for the parking. Ange likes her food, bless her. All was well until I stood in the queue to pay and spotted, to my horror, a pregnant woman at the next checkout. I quickly grabbed my stuff and got away from there, thinking she would never know how close she had come to giving birth there and then in Waitrose. I know their logo is green, but I'm not sure even they would appreciate a glowing green radioactive baby clogging up their checkout aisle.

Second Procedure

The next procedure I had was a laparoscopy, which I was told was a minor operation under general anaesthetic (much better than sergeant sedation), where they make a small incision in the naval and inflate your abdomen with carbon dioxide. This is a keyhole-type surgery and allows the surgeon to see the size and spread of the tumour and surrounding area, without carving you like a turkey at Christmas. Mine was done at Maidstone Hospital. I turned up on the appointed day and again was handed a lovely dressing-gown and some surgical socks (no suspenders, though!) There is something levelling about a room full of people all looking slightly apprehensive in their gowns and socks; unless of course you have had diabetic problems, and they needed to give you only one sock!

One thing that was consistent with me was that, every time I had an operation or procedure, for some reason I thought it was very important for me to ensure that my bowel area was completely poo free. No-one had ever told me that I must go for a no.2 prior to these procedures, but I just had a feeling that when they sliced into me the last thing a highly trained surgeon needed was the remains of my digestive system squirted across his features. 'Wipe, please, nurse!' Well, this again confirms to you my lack of medical knowledge, but for some reason I was convinced it would save me huge amounts of embarrassment.

There is a mental foundation for this, tenuous I know, but, hey, it's my psyche. A few years ago I had to undergo circumcision at the grand age of forty-four, I think it was. This was a result of some issues with my diabetes. As mentioned earlier with the one-stocking hand-out, diabetes can lead to serious issues, including the amputation of limbs. Now I shan't be so boastful as to say the surgeon performing my circumcision was going to have to remove a foot, but you know how we men like to boast! Anyway, the point is that, after the surgery, I was moving from the trolley used to transport me back to the ward-bed, and, as I looked down, all I could see was brown, brown and more brown. I panicked in the way only Bill Clinton could have done when he was offered a box of Cuban cigars by a congressional investigator and was just about to break down in sobs of 'I'm so sorry,' when the nurse with me pointed out that it was in fact iodine that had been used, and it wasn't my bottom reverting to its six-month-old state. Relieved? I could have paid my TV licence. So now you see why my mind had convinced me to evacuate all chances of embarrassment prior to any procedures and why I very nearly missed my slot to be operated on, as, while the nurse was trying to locate me, I was in a toilet squeezing harder than a Del Monte orange-packer.

As with a lot of these procedures, there is bound to be a bit of pain on your waking, and a laparoscopy is definitely one. I woke in the recovery-room and was just getting my bearings when it felt like someone was trying to pull my arm from its socket, and I wailed like a small child who's just realised that the biggest present under the Christmas tree is for his sister. (Yeah, got that one in, Shirley!) Apparently the carbon dioxide gas they use to inflate you (makes a huge change from getting deflated about it all) needs to escape from your body cavity, and for some reason it heads to your shoulder area, much like a moth to a light. I cannot understand the medical reason for this, as I don't recall having an outlet valve in my armpit, but it has something to do with your diaphragm muscle and its connection to your shoulder muscle, I believe, but again don't quote me. Anyway, the lovely nurse looking after me gauged my waking reaction quicker than Mr Bolt getting to his next gold medal, and I was given some morphine. Now I've done my homework here (ha, lazy-minded, indeed!), and I must give praise to Friedrich Sertürner who back in 1804 discovered this wonderful drug. I am aware that it can cause its own issues if overused, but I have had it on many occasions in the past months, and every time it has been as needed as a huge box of Dairy Milk by a recently dumped-again spinster.

So, back in the recovery room, the morphine was numbing the pain like the mute button on a bad X-Factor audition, and I had a chance to look at my first set of operation scars. For reasons best known to the surgeon, he had made three incisions in me: the first, as advised, on my belly-button and two further ones each about an inch below my nipples, making me look as if I had a big smiley face on my torso. Perhaps they needed a lot more gas, and therefore more access to get it into me, in order to lift my not insubstantial outer casing.

Well, as the pain subsided, I was taken up to a recovery-ward and, after initial checks, I was left on my own and ignored for a couple of hours. By this time I was quite hungry and was given the option of a sandwich or a biscuit. Now as I have mentioned, since I was having great trouble eating bread, a sandwich was out if the question. 'Is there any soup at all or any other option, please?' I asked the ward-assistant. 'Sorry, no, so which would you like?' I settled for a small pack of three (bourbons, that is) while contemplating the fact I was really hungry. The smell of the food being consumed by the patients in the ward opposite drifted towards me. 'Shepherd's pie,' I thought, while remembering a part in the pre-procedure literature that said I must eat before leaving the hospital.

I went home feeling desperate just to get back to the solitude of my own flat. The bourbons still lay on my bedside tray back in the recovery-ward. I was picked up by Colin, my manager from work, who along with the rest of work had been very supportive of me, and, as I got into his car, I was handed a bag of presents from my colleagues, which included various bags of crisps, biscuits and sausage-rolls. So their timing was perfect, and I looked forward to getting home and munching with aplomb. It was my birthday a couple of days later, and I sat there singing *Happy Birthday to Me* into a mirror, wondering which I should hate most: the cancer; the surgeon who booked a procedure so close to my festive day; or the subsequent discomfort that discouraged me from even contemplating celebrating in any shape. I settled on all three and really felt empathy for old misunderstood Ebenezer Scrooge. I must add that I received a call from a sister at the hospital a day or so later, and I did discuss with her the dietary options available post-op, and she agreed that something like soup would be a good thing to have. Eat your heart out, James Martin.

Third Procedure

My final procedure, a while later, was an endoscopic ultrasound. Unfortunately this wasn't Midge Ure and his gang singing Vienna to me; it is sound pulses that give the operator a picture of the size and spread in more detail than the other procedures. Mine was back at QEQM. By this time, Ange had got ordering the breakfast option in the hospital canteen down to a T. I feel proud of how I supported her by ensuring my plate was made up to the allotted seven items by adding things I could not eat but which coincidentally she just happened to like.

This procedure was done by a surgeon, and, as I was escorted into the room, I couldn't help but notice the plethora of people in white coats hovering around me. All my endoscopic procedures so far had been done under the warm blanket of mild sedation. This is a bit more than a local anaesthetic, but you are not as completely out of it as with a general anaesthetic. Now my first endoscopy was pretty much pain-free, so I wasn't expecting this one to be any different. Oh, how wrong I was! I could feel the movement inside. Whether that was the probe or the ultrasound I still do not know, but I was pretty sure I looked like John Hurt after eating a Chinese meal whilst a small creature rummaged around under his skin. I have a theory that the surgeon let the other white-coated bodies in the room have a go on me, like a giant real live version of the game Operation, but I cannot be sure because with sedation you feel the pain but are still pretty much out of things. I was initially told, by whom I cannot recall, that you cannot have a general anaesthetic for an endoscopic procedure because they need you to be able to swallow, which made sense to me. I have, however, found out that this is not the case and you can have a general, but on the whole I would suggest you go with the doctors' or surgeons' advice, unless you are likely to panic like an arachnophobe in the cupboard under the stairs on a moist summer evening.

*****

Well, that was the three procedures now done, and, as I said previously, the aim was to ascertain the general shape, size and spread of my individual tumour by staging my cancer. Now, I had been given a slight heads-up by the lovely morphine-administering nurse in the recovery-room after my laparoscopy, in that the surgeon had left the papers with his findings with me, and I was allowed to see that, after the procedure, he viewed my cancer as stage T4 N2 MO. Now this may as well have been written in Klingon for all the sense it made to me, but at least I now had a number. What it means is three separate things. T4 means that the cancer has grown into other body areas. N2 means that there is cancer in three-to-six lymph nodes nearby, and MO states that there has been no cancer spread to other organs.

At this point I must say that it is extremely important that you do not take this as the rule for all. This is what I was advised, and this relates specifically to me, so it cannot be interpreted without confirmation to fit all. I'm saying that it really would not be fair of me to deprive you of the wonderful joyous experience of having your own procedures done so that your own conclusions can be found. There was no dramatic announcement of my stage at any meeting I can recall. The information I gleaned was through being copied in on letters to my GP and searches on the internet.

I feel at this point that I must advise extreme caution if you do decide to type into 'tinternet' whatever diagnosis you may have, because, trust me: you will see more sites with pieces of conflicting information than a habitual eater sees McDonald's wrappers. When I got home after first being diagnosed, I succumbed to the natural curiosity we all have and put into my search engine 'oesophageal cancer' and watched the many sites roll by. Well, after a few minutes of looking, I discovered that I only had a 20% chance of survival and about six months to live. Before I bolted for the Bacardi bottle, I thought I would check a little more closely and discovered that, yes, the survival rate was correct … if I was a male in his late seventies, who had been diagnosed after giving the cancer time to leisurely lunch around his vital organs for several years, and was as weak as a kitten that had spent several days playing dress-up with Marjorie Malone, the odious kid from the next street. I wasn't, I hadn't and Marjorie doesn't exist, but the point is that information on the internet is at best vague and at worst misleading. It can be a handy tool for checking details on official NHS websites, such as procedures and staging, as I have already mentioned, but it can also scare you worse than a winter electricity bill when you realise you've left the upstairs two-bar heater on for the past three months. So by all means look, but always remember that each case is individual. You are an individual, so you cannot be a generic set of symptoms. The NHS professionals will answer you. You may not like the answer, and you may have to chase, but that is what they are there for.

The next step in my case was to have an appointment with my oncologist, Dr Waters: a very agreeable man in a very challenging job. Well, that is the way I see his position. There are many jobs that people undertake in the professional healthcare world that touch death, and I would imagine the chance to change that option for a patient was motivation enough for these people, but to deal with it constantly is a calling that I believe only some can truly master in a caring, professional and understanding way. Not everyone you meet will have these attributes, despite their working closely with such cases, but the ones that do will make you understand a little better why it takes a certain type of person to be a good healthcare worker. Dr Waters was such a person. He came across as very knowledgeable, sympathetic, understanding, honest and, above all ... Ange fancied him! So I discussed with the good doctor the past tests and procedures while Ange swooned like a vapid teen at a One D concert. Band? The only band on stage there is the one holding the zit cream to the mike stand - session musicians excluded, of course!

Now up until this point I had been under the impression that the containment of the tumour looked good, and, as long as it was all centralised in one area, the operation would be going ahead. In between the procedures, I had been given an appointment to meet my main surgeon, Professor Nisar, at Maidstone Hospital, for a discussion of the main operation to be performed, if the tumour did prove operable. Is it just me, or does the word 'professor' alone not fill you with confidence and respect? That is, until you remember Professor Pat Pending from the Wacky Races or Professor Chaos aka Butters for the South Park fans. Well, I met my soon-to-be-future surgeon. Oh, how things change! But more on that coming up, folks.

The operation was explained to me. Apparently the oesophagectomy is one of the major and most invasive procedures currently performed in the UK. I should be slit from throat to abdomen and peeled back like a banana skin;

the offending items would be located and disposed of like the baddies in an espionage film. Slight melodrama used, but hey-ho, it's my body and my book! The main point made was that, because it was such a major operation, it would be done only if they believed beforehand that they would be able to remove all the cancer in one go. There would be no attempt at proportional extraction. It was like the Small Faces song: *All or Nothing*. Now is it me, or does proportional extraction sound like the next political debate the SDP will be having? The plan, therefore, was for me to have chemotherapy to shrink the tumour, making the surgery easier with a better chance of success.

Well, I discussed the findings with Ange's love-interest doctor. (May I just take this opportunity to state, for the sake of Ange's boyfriend, that she in no way made moves on the good doctor, and, for the sake of Mrs Waters, if there is one, that, as far as I am aware, Dr Waters had no idea of this infatuation. I believe he just assumed the odd sigh and the damp patches came from my emotional inability to deal with things.) The vast majority of the discussion confirmed the original scan findings in that the cancer was limited to the tumour and a few nodes in my stomach close to it.

The tumour, now a healthy 11cm long and fast approaching teenage years (I wondered whether tumours get zits), was contained. It had started recruiting but hadn't as yet gathered an army - a bit like UKIP. (Quite like the idea of using them in reference to an invading body!) The issue, however, was that the ultrasound test had discovered that the width of the tumour, and how it was attached to the surrounding anatomy, was a little deeper than initially thought. What this meant was that the chemotherapy now being discussed was a little more important than I had originally thought. I knew that shrinking the tumour was important for the surgery and that chemotherapy would hopefully do that and halt the little bugger from trying to be a dictator and invade Heartsville or Lungtown. What was now sinking in was that, if the chemo didn't work to the point of shrinking this newly-discovered girth of my tumour, I should be back to that wonderful word 'palliative', as they would not operate. It's amazing how the word 'girth' had made me chuckle over the years, but it now took on a complete new sense of impotence; no pun intended.

Chapter Six

Emotional Stuff

If you have managed never to be dragged to a roller-coaster and cajoled into one of its seats to be given the 'ride of your life,' then I'm afraid this chapter is going to be a bit of a shocker, as the ride you are about to take is probably one of the most real, extreme and relentless you will ever have; but at least it's free. The biggest difference is that, with a diagnosis of cancer, there is no five-minute calm 'chug' to the top before gravity takes its hold and propels you through as many different types of acting forces as is possible; or as the local council will allow you. Quite simply, one minute you are doing whatever you are doing, and then everything changes. I have expelled more liquid from my nose than Oliver Reed could drink. I have shed more tears in one hour than the entire cast of Eastenders on a Christmas special, and I have been in places that felt darker than a fifty-year-old virgin's special parts. The biggest problem with all of these is that they can come from absolutely nowhere, with no warning or reason.

Being a 'British Chap' I and my emotions have always led a kind of accepted dance throughout my life. I knew they were there, and they could occasionally embarrass me. Just as long as they generally kept themselves in check and didn't cause me any major grief, I was happy to let them live in that little box I had created for them. Ironically, though, I am quite an emotional type of person, being the son of a musician with ability in the dramatic arts at school and all whilst being forced to sit through regular sessions of old black-and-white films on a Sunday afternoon. Well, I say 'forced' ... I guess the first inkling I may have had with this particular aspect of nature-nurture was when I joined the RAF at seventeen: full of emotions, all having to be suppressed and controlled - which is not a bad thing, but the inner excitable child was always trying to pop out and say hello. Now that can be quite difficult when you're carrying a sub-machine-gun with live ammunition because a certain USA president decides to bomb a certain African so-called dictator, using the country I was posted to as a refuelling post - quite ironic when you consider he probably based his decision on his emotions. But that night I came pretty close to being wiped out whilst stoically trying to contain mine; but then I am only writing a book, so the American psyche and its emotions definitely wouldn't fit. This is becoming repetitive, but all I can say in this chapter, as with all the others, is that, again, this is very much an individual thing. Some people can go through their entire lives without breaking an emotional sweat. Some snap more quickly than a Thatcher U-turn: oh, yes, she did.

What I have found in general life, and again I am no expert, is that the chemical balance in our bodies directly affects the emotional balance we feel during normal life. I think this is why some people cry harder, laugh longer, hug more tightly and break more easily than others. It is not a 'head-problem' in my understanding: it is a balance problem. Take depression (please, take it Mr Marx). The way I see it is that we fall into a trough where we cannot see over the side, and therefore we cannot see a way beyond the trough. I believe that for most with a normal chemical balance there comes the point where the view is revealed beyond the trough, and we see the route out, and on we go. Some, however, can get stuck in that trough for a very long time. Some can be allowed to see a way out only for it to be obscured from them just as they try to extricate themselves. I would be silly and wrong to suggest I can try to explain any aspect that encroaches on mental health issues, but this is just a general interpretation I have about certain aspects, based on dealing with my own issues and problems over the years and through knowing people who have had to deal with much greater problems. The point I am trying to make here is that, again, it is an individual thing, and, although I can tell you about my problems, any solutions for yourself will have to come from you. Obviously someone's diagnosing you with cancer is quite an emotional thing. If you don't react in an emotional way to that at some point, you may as well buy yourself a really good snorkel and go settle with all the other molluscs in the rock-pool down on the seafront; or, if you live inland, just join a call-centre selling PPI or the like. As I said at the start of this book, I went from total denial to disbelief, to acceptance of the inevitable, in two days. Cancer is one of those things that hover on the periphery of most people's lives. Most have been touched by it in one way or another, and unfortunately this seems to be on the increase. It is like a car crash that you pass on the motorway: you know they happen, and, as the lottery publicity says, 'It could be you,' but you have this inner belief that it will always be some other poor bugger. When the big finger does point at you, the realisation of what it entails is sometimes too vast for us to comprehend immediately, and I believe that we will always go through certain stages to allow the information to be properly assimilated.

For me, as I have said, the immediate issue was not really of the fight ahead: it was more an initial thought of whether I really wanted to beat it. This may seem very negative and obtuse, but we all know that, as life rolls over us, certain things happen that make us ask big questions of ourselves, and looking death in the face like a strange head-to-head episode of *Alas Smith & Jones* is probably one of the most important. 'Life is what happens when you're busy making other plans,' said Mr Lennon, and I believe that is very true, but occasionally the plans and life come into direct conflict with each other - a bit like a politician and his policies. So the question I was facing was quite simply, 'Did I want to survive?' The reason behind this for me was based on inevitability. I have always rolled with the punches, so to speak. Whenever life threw me a curve ball, I just accepted it and moved along the deviated path that seemed to have been chosen for me. I guess that could be going back to my being 'lazy-minded', or it could be that I believed in a Higher Power helping me with the tougher decisions and gently nudging me in the right direction. Either way, I pretty much always accepted things that happened to me with a sort of benign motivation: a bit like Cheryl Cole's career, except that I have the greatest of respect for people who choose to look after my coat. Here, however, was the biggest choice I had ever been faced with. Do I face this beast as everyone would expect me to, or do I accept that everything happens for a reason and perhaps this was something that was meant to be?

I know some will not get in any way what I was even considering, but, as I have said, this is personal to me. I mention it because I do believe that some will have the same thoughts during their personal road-trip to hell and back. This also wasn't just a fleeting thought that came and went like a one-night stand in Ayia Napa (gosh, I had some fun out there!): this was something that chewed away at me for weeks. What changed my perception, however, and convinced me that this wasn't meant to be my swan-song was this: at the same time as my diagnosis, there occurred that awful tragedy where the train crashed in Spain. Those poor souls were just commuting or holidaying, and bang: gone! If I was meant to be leaving this majestic planet that's evolving or revolving at 900mph (sorry, Python again), surely something like that would happen to me. So I decided in my mind that I would not go quietly into that dark night. I'd write some lyrics about it; kick myself up the arse and be grateful for what I had; and use the opportunity to take this bugger on and see where I ended up. The way I did it (and it is what got me through some pretty dark times) was to focus on the next stage. After diagnosis I focused on the spread and the tests to establish that. Then I focused on the chemotherapy, then whether it was operable, and so on, until I got to the end one way or another. Great song, and how Blondie did it for me; thanks for killing that ID.

I guess the hardest thing to deal with going through all this is that you can be chugging along quite content in what is happening, and all of a sudden you will be weeping more than Bridget Jones watching the last episode of *Friends*. This can happen at any time and can be triggered by almost anything. Many times I would be just sitting watching the telly when I would feel an overriding sense of loss and bewilderment and just start leaking like a tap with a broken washer. I did not always know where it came from and just had to let it happen. Quite a few times, though, something will happen in your treatments or procedures that will remind you of exactly where you are, and you react as if you have been hit by a sledgehammer and are reduced to a whimpering fool. I have no idea whether this is normal, although I have been told it is, and I believe that the most important thing is how we react to these situations. A couple of times in the early days, this happened to me, and I reacted in the only way I could think of. I went into the kitchen, grabbed a bottle of Bacardi and proceeded to pour drinks only just smaller than the bottle itself. I could lie here and say this was incredibly unhelpful and stupid, but the truth is, I usually had only one or two and quite frankly they helped me calm down and relax. I don't know whether it was because it took my mind to somewhere more fuzzy or because it made me look at myself and what I was doing, but for me it did help on those couple of occasions. I don't advocate going and getting rip-roaring drunk every time you have an issue through your treatment, otherwise there would be a serious world booze shortage and poor genuine tramps would struggle to keep up their state-paid intake of liquid abuse. However, a little of what gets you through can't be all that bad. I would suggest that, if you are a heroin-addicted sex-worker, you should really stave off any binge impulses. The point for me was that I could be knocked sideways emotionally by nothing or something, and I had to find a way of getting things back on to an even keel.

One of the biggest issues for me, which would help the little tear gremlins, was a sense of isolation. I know I have great friends, but I don't have a partner, so for 95% of my time dealing with this illness I was pretty much alone. This isn't said for the 'aah' factor, because, as I have said before, I was pretty well supported by friends and family. The only trouble was that they were not with me on a day-to-day basis as a partner would have been. I like to think that I am still single because my devastating looks and voracious sexual appetite tend to scare potential partners away. The truth is that I've been a bit of an idiot and let past experiences and petty insecurities stop me from having a relationship, on more than one occasion. So here I was alone, but sort of OK with it. However, that doesn't stop your wanting that personal intimacy of shared feelings at the time you most need it. The most difficult thing was that occasionally I would find myself moaning at friends just because they were the substitute for a partner. Some were fine with it, but some couldn't cope, especially when you consider that this wasn't a couple of weeks of trauma but months of drawn-out issues. I cannot blame them, as it must have been difficult listening to Victor Meldrew banging on about poor old him, but it was the only form of release I had, and many times I ended up relieved I had vented my spleen but also very down because it had caused a rift between myself and a friend.

Therein lies one of the biggest issues you will have to face through your treatments and dealings with cancer: you will worry more about others close to you than you do about yourself. If you don't, just pull your slacks up to your chin and press your red buzzer. I am not sure whether what I went through was a normal emotional path, as everything about it is, again, specific to your problems and personality, but I feel that I just about kept things together on several occasions, and I got to the other side of each episode just about intact, like watching *The Office*, and I think if you can manage to achieve that you're doing pretty well. A few times I did feel that I was sinking lower than J Lo's butt and really did consider biting the bullet and asking for help, but owing to my stubborn attitude based on the previous dealings with so-called counsellors, I decided against it. My only advice to you is just to use every option available to you. Don't be proud and British, use the support-mechanisms around you and keep your head above the water, no matter what it takes.

As I have said in the chapter dealing with the NHS, I have come across some truly remarkable and fantastic people in the NHS, and one such that made me re-think things about counselling was my specialist nurse, Sue. It was as I was approaching the end of my chemotherapy and I had an appointment with my oncologist and we knew what was coming in: that there was an extremely high likelihood of my getting my all-clear. This was based on the fact that, with my specific cancer and path of treatment, the main operation would not have been attempted if they didn't believe that they could get all the cancer; and the indications post-op were very encouraging. This is where the experience and knowledge of specialists will help you greatly, as Sue realised: this was a time when lots of patients can feel very isolated and almost abandoned. Once you are in the position of being all-clear, the mechanisms around you start to peel away more quickly than a pickpocket's hand on a crowded tube. So Sue had pre-empted me on this, and she was absolutely correct. The strangest thing is seeing every person around you celebrate and pop the champagne, but in your heart of hearts all you feel is confused and lost. So I did what John Wayne would have done, bit the bullet and made an appointment to see a counsellor; fortunately not the same one from my earlier experience, which you will discover later.

I found the experience quite strange, and again it is very much down to the individual's personal circumstances and willingness to attempt to communicate their experience and feelings, but there was a lot of waffling from me and some very salient points from the lovely lady who was listening to me with more patience than all the saints at the Last Supper combined - even in a Dan Brown book. I found that it helped me to put more perspective on the experiences I had and also how I had dealt with them, and also it assisted me in putting a form of sense and order to events, a bit like some strange cerebral library Dewey system. For example, the abandonment I felt on my getting what should have been fantastic news over my all-clear made perfect sense when you consider that I had been focusing on the next stage up until then, and all of a sudden there was no next stage. What I didn't think of was that when your brain deals with such a huge sensory overload, such as being diagnosed, it will go into an automatic state of logical progression, like focusing on the next thing, almost like a fight-or-flight response. It does this the better to process the situation and help you deal with it, but when you get to the point of the roller-coaster's ending, you revert to normal function, and all of a sudden all the realisations and feelings you thought were under check are suddenly free to wander about your psyche like some depraved Bonnie and Clyde out to cause as much havoc as possible. What I took from all of this was to be prepared, to understand and sometimes to accept but also to realise that it is all very normal - you just didn't know it. I do, however go into more detail on this later in the book.

The only thing I can really say in this chapter is that you will go through more than you think you can handle. You will have extreme feelings about, and towards, the people closest to you. You will worry more than an agoraphobic in the desert, and it may take more time than you envisaged or hoped, but you can get there. Ask for help if you need it. Take support when it's offered, and remember that those that love you still love you.

Chapter Seven

Family and Friends

Once again, how people around you deal with your diagnosis and treatment is an individual thing. Obviously it is a huge blow to all when you first find out that you have the dreaded C, and different people will react in different ways. As I said before, I had always hoped that, if it ever did happen to me, I should be able to keep it to myself and deal with it quietly, but that was not going to happen. When you do tell people, it will be very hard for them to comprehend things, and the only thing I can suggest is that you are totally honest from the start and allow them the time they need to absorb this information. I personally found it difficult to tell those closest to me, because I felt in some strange way that I was putting a burden on them and making them feel they were now part of something that they also didn't deserve. Most people I told were initially obviously quite shocked and needed time to let it sink in, just as I had. I think it is a time to bring out the politician in you: I don't mean start roaming well-known commons and fiddling your work expenses, as if it were a free day at the sweet-shop. I mean, get the information clear in your head and choose your words carefully. I know this will be difficult, but don't forget, there is no manual or procedure list for this. Just remember, they care about you and will understand, eventually.

The difficulty I found is the different reactions you will get from some. This news will have a serious impact on your relationships, and you have to accept that some people deal with things like this better than others. That does not make people good or bad; it's just down to individual coping mechanisms. Some will try and smother you with kindness, whereas some will need to keep a certain distance from you emotionally in order to cope. You cannot forget that cancer is so prevalent nowadays that most people you know will have been touched by it; some may even have lost people close to them because of it. The most important thing I have found is not to judge or make any rash decisions about people. Don't forget that even though this is happening to you, they are suffering just as much and dealing with it the only way they know how. The worst thing that you can do is to make any rash or judgemental decisions, because things done at emotionally charged moments can do more damage than a frustrated wife with a platinum credit-card. After all, the aim is to beat your illness and regain your previous life, so getting there, but losing people close to you, is a hollow victory. You will find, as the news of your illness leaks into your social stratum, that some people will find it difficult to be around you, or even to have a conversation with you. This is not because cancer suddenly gives you halitosis or body-odour: it is just that some simply cannot deal with it. Just remember, it is the cancer they cannot cope with, not you. I found the easiest way to deal with this kind of situation was simply to laugh it off. I will not lie: there are times in dealing with people (some very close to me) when you feel angry and hurt that the reaction you are getting is not what you had hoped for or expected from them, but just remember, this is affecting them as well, and nothing about this lovely disease is easy or straightforward. The one thing I found (and this is no judgement on anyone) is that some people close to you that you expected more from often provided less, but some you expected nothing from often provided the most. That is the great thing about people: they constantly surprise you. The thing I found myself doing a lot was trying to put myself in their shoes: what should I do if the roles were reversed? The trouble with that is, you often feel that you would have done things better, so therefore you feel as if that person failed you, especially when your name is Saint Quinn of Bacardi.

The truth is that no one person does exactly the same thing as everyone else, even in the exact same circumstances. To my mind, this means that you can never judge someone as a person basing your judgement on just one event. To be positive about my personal situation, I should say that there were things friends did that warmed me more quickly than a large brandy on a cold day; or, as I described, more quickly that the injection during a CT scan. And these things not only made dealing with things a lot easier, but also reminded me that some people do care quite a lot about me.

There was Ange, who was with me at diagnosis. She decided there and then, I guess, that as well as taking me to as many of my appointments prior to my main operation as she could (after which I managed to secure patient transport), I should also receive a 'morning hug' text every day. She also became very proficient at listening to me whilst I vented my spleen like a dog with a sore paw. (That reminds me of one of my father's favourite jokes. A dog limps into a saloon with a bandaged foot, looks at the barman and says, 'I've come for the guy that shot ma paw'! Sorry, that does make me chuckle.) I often felt that I put too much on Ange, but bless her, she never said No to a vent; was always supportive; and reminded me of exactly what I was going through and the fact that it was quite a big deal and I wasn't doing too badly. But more importantly to me, she had the ability to be this great support whilst remaining honest and objective. She did, however, let me down on several occasions when her boyfriend came over and they demolished several bottles of wine and went on to some serious snuggling – but, hey, I forgive you, hun, lol!

My sister also blew me away with her determination and support. A month or so after my being diagnosed, she and my bother-in-law Dom decided that it was time for them to come and visit me. It was well overdue, regardless of my diagnosis, but I pretty much knew from talking to her that the main reason for her visit was for her to satisfy herself that I was well-supported and in a position to get through whatever lay ahead. As it happened, she met nearly all my friends and could see I was doing OK, so we decided to have the most rip-roaring booze-fuelled couple of days since a boat-load of whisky washed up off the coast of Scotland. Again, Shirley was a constant support throughout it all, and one of the most emotional days I recently had was when I was able to visit Shirley just after my all-clear, and support her whilst she and some colleagues from work did the Race for Life in Nottingham. It was very poignant when I was able to open a rather nice bottle of champagne that my MD had given me as an all-clear gift and share it with these lovely ladies, after they completed the race. I was so emotional I very nearly didn't have a good stare at these gorgeous young ladies and contemplate a new job in Nottingham. Not that there are not lots of lovely ladies in my company … I think I had better stop there.

My cousins and friends have been very supportive to me, but there comes a point, as already mentioned, where things can get stale or awkward. This can be down to treatments, their perspective, putting too much pressure on them, or a combination. One of the things I did from the very start of my treatment was to send a message out regularly to certain family and friends, just updating them on the latest bit of information (almost as the kind people at CNN do for the American government). I would try to make it light, positive and informative, but in my mind I felt as if I was keeping them in the loop and involved in the situation. Also, this information would usually trickle out from these people to others, saving me lots of updating if and when I bumped into people, and it was especially good at keeping people in touch that could not get to see me for reasons of either work or distance.

What I found was that at first I would be inundated with responses and positive replies, but then, as time dragged on and the months passed, the responses would become less and less frequent, sort of like the conversation at breakfast after a new partner moves in. I took this to mean that people were perhaps starting to wonder whether my situation was ever going to end. Again - I keep repeating it - cancers and your treatment are unique. Some cancers will be sorted in a matter of weeks, and some may go on for years. I believe that the biggest issue for people on your periphery that are going through it as well is that they have their own lives to deal with as well as the insecurity of dealing with you. In my own case I believe that, because things were taking the time they did to get from one stage to the next - just because of the way my treatment had to happen - that people had no normality, and that is why eventually they began to struggle. And as time went by, this sense of uncertainty was difficult for others to absorb into their day-to-day lives. If, however, the assessments and treatments leading to the end-result had been more compressed, that might have helped. I know of people who have had very quick positive dealings with cancer, and that is obviously great for all concerned. I also know people who have had dealings with cancer that have lasted years, and even in these cases I think that, once the initial understanding of the prognosis is sorted and the treatment is under way, there is a return to an (approximate) form of normality, even in awful situations. Again, each case will be different, and again, all I can say is that the most important thing to try to achieve is to beat this bugger of a disease and get your life back, preferably with the same people you had at the start still being around without wanting constantly to throttle you.

One of the biggest helps to me in my year with this lovely bundle of joy called cancer was the way my company assisted me throughout the whole of my treatment. The initial shockwave that went round the company when I told them and the responses I had from people I had worked with for almost ten years was heartfelt and genuine - apart from Mr Grimley, the car-park attendant, but he still hadn't forgiven the last department of pesky kids who had thwarted his plans to steal the Hope Diamond. I was lucky enough to work for a company that was sufficiently large to be in a position to keep my job open and me on the payroll. They also have an ethos of looking after long-term staff, as they understand that they are the company's biggest investment. More than that, I really felt that there was a genuine understanding from my MD down, that they knew it was simply the right thing to do. Not only did I receive as much time as I needed for hospital appointments and treatments: I was also actively encouraged to listen to my doctors and do exactly as they advised.

Anyone who is unfortunate enough to go through something like this will understand that nowadays we don't all have savings to fall back on, and the simple fact is that, if I had not kept my job, I should definitely have lost my flat. And who knows what else may have happened which could only have had a negative effect on my health, both emotional and physical? One of the most supportive things that my own office did for me, as well as giving emotional support, was that some of my team would go out of their way daily to give me lifts to and from work. What I tried to do, once I understood the plan for my treatment, was to minimise the time off work. As I knew that the time off after my operation would be considerable (up to six months, I had been advised), I tried to minimise this by taking as little time as needed in 2013 leading up to the operation. This was something I did myself, and I managed it, although sometimes I was instructed by my company to take a few more days than I had planned to. In the end, during the first few months, I managed to do as much as I could, but many times this involved me going in early and working till I couldn't carry on. Then I would go home, but at least I felt I was doing something, and most times I was doing a high percentage of the hours I was required to do. I must emphasise, though, that I was very lucky, because during this period the only person putting pressure on me to do the hours I was doing was myself.

One thing that happened a couple of months after my operation was that I was advised by my HR manager – a supportive lady called Cherrie - that the company's insurance company would be giving me a call. I was quite keen on this, because it meant that the company would get some remuneration for my pay. Anyway, the lady from the insurance company called a few days later and asked whether we could have a chat about my illness and what the prognosis was. I went through some of the things that had been happening and the hoped-for plan for the coming months. It was only when I heard the lump forming in the lady's voice that I asked her whether she was OK. She admitted that she usually dealt only with people with bad backs and 'nervous' issues and was feeling quite upset by what I had gone through and was going through. I then knew the insurance company wouldn't be contesting any claim my company was making. At this point I felt more relieved than George Michael after a trip to a public convenience. Again, not because my company was putting any pressure on me, but it alleviated the pressure I was putting on myself in my own mind. As it happened in my case, the recovery went over the six-month period, mainly due to the many extra procedures and hospital stays I had after my main operation, but again my company were very supportive. The main thing that we all wanted to happen was for me to be back to work in a position where I was able and capable of doing my job. This involved a gradual staged return where I worked only mornings for the first couple of weeks, but the goal was for me to move forward in my return and not to have any setbacks that would hinder my recovery.

Chapter Eight

Chemotherapy

My chemotherapy was due to start towards the end of September. After a discussion with Dr Waters, the plan for me was to have three types: E, C and X. Two of these would be administered intravenously, and the third would be in the form of a course of tablets. I would have a day in the chemotherapy unit at QEQM, Margate, and take the tablets at home, along with all my other medication. I was beginning to rattle as I walked by this point, but it would save me using the tambourine if I did any gigs. It was a course of three cycles (don't panic, no exercise required) of treatment and was timed so that the next treatment would begin as the previous course of tablets ended. I should love to be able to give a detailed description of what each of the drugs is and what it does, but I am not that knowledgeable. However, I do know that the E is for Epirubican, and this is the one that causes the hair-loss. The truth is that there are quite a few types, again dependent on the type of cancer being treated, so the cocktail given is very much designed for the individual. My cocktail, I later discovered, was quite intense and should be called 'Slowly being screwed whilst leaning against the wall'!

Roughly two days prior to any chemotherapy treatments, you have to visit the unit so they can assess your fitness, weigh you and so that blood can be taken and checked. I always found this quite a pain, as it usually took about twenty minutes. It seemed to me that it could have been done by my giving blood and being physically checked at my doctor's surgery; if required, I could have had a chat with the chemotherapy nurse over the phone. Alas, the system will not allow this excessive use of common sense, and you must present yourself for full inspection at the allotted time. I don't mean to be obtuse when I mention this, but there are many times I have had 'pointless' appointments during my treatment. As I have described, I am not a retired person with a car and time, so that I can just potter over to have a chat. I was at this time still trying to be at work as much as possible (the office may disagree), and, although taking the time to go from work was not an issue, arranging transport etc. was. As with lots of my appointments, I was very much reliant on the help of others. Ange, work and lots of friends were very supportive, and they would give me lifts whenever they could, but they were working, too, and it usually meant time off for them; but more on this later.

Well prior to the chemotherapy treatments' starting, I had an appointment with Dr Waters in which all the possible side-effects and problems that might arise were outlined. The list is quite frankly as scary as the Hammer House of Horror movies were to me when I was about ten. (For those that don't remember, they were bloody terrifying.) There are about fifteen major side-effects and about twenty minor ones. As he ticked the boxes that may affect me, based on the drugs I was to be given, and handed me the paperwork, I looked down and noticed the only box he hadn't ticked was 'Early Menopause'. I wasn't sure whether I was disappointed because I couldn't tick the last box, which would give me the right to leap in the air and shout 'bingo!', or because it was all suddenly becoming very real.

The very first occasion you have your two-day pre-check is more involved, and mine duly arrived. I met the nurse who was going to take me through the treatment, and we went through various points relative to my condition and then moved on to the chemotherapy itself. The important thing to bear in mind with the side-effects that keep getting mentioned is that they are, as they tell you, possible but not certain. As with many aspects of this disease, it will affect different people in different ways: it is unique to the individual case. I think that the reason you keep getting these side-effects drummed into you is, firstly, so that you can be aware, but also because I believe that we are increasingly becoming a society that exists in the good ol' USA way of lawsuits: 'Mum, I burned my lip on this apple pie!' Kerrrching! Therefore I felt that there was a certain amount of self-protection in the constant advice being given; I may be wrong, but that's how it felt to me.

Cutting through all the reams of possible side-effects I might have, it boiled down to two things they were concerned about. You are given a book with lots of information about things that might come up after treatment whilst at home and what to do and whom to contact over them, but there are two things that should raise a red flag (neither is Russian), and they are diarrhoea and sickness. If either one of these lasts for more than a day, you must ring up and seek advice. One more thing is to buy yourself a thermometer, as the first thing you will be asked for if you call is your temperature. The only real advice I can give here and throughout treatment is to hold back your initial thoughts until you have all the facts. I say this because sometimes we react to a statement, and our initial line of thinking may not be the quite the line meant. For example, the nurse discussed with me the point of hair-loss. Now I know that she was simply going from the 'script', but one glance at my head should have made her realise that my head was as barren as the Gobi Desert, and losing hair wasn't exactly a worry to me. The only thing I was quite miffed about was that I had, only a few weeks previously, bought myself a new set of hair-trimmers to tidy up the odd hair that managed to fight its way out. However, she discussed it, and one point she made was that she had seen many ladies who were quite obviously nervous about this aspect of the chemotherapy and I suppose, to lighten the mood, they had asked her whether it was just the hair on their heads that would be affected. My initial instinct was to make a joke about Brazilians or runways, but I held back just long enough for the nurse to say, 'Well, I tell them, sorry, but you will still have to keep shaving your legs!' So, as I say, wait till all the facts are in.

Two days later, I found myself sitting outside the chemotherapy unit as nervous as a teenage girl waiting for the pregnancy-test to dry and decide her fate. The ward itself is just a large room with a dozen reclining chairs (no beds) in little bay-type areas; a central nurses' station; and lots of bleeping noises. I was allocated my bay, and my arm was wrapped in a heating blanket to make finding my veins slightly easier than finding Lord Lucan. The one thing I hated that first day was that the bay they had put me in was right by the nurses' station. Now I didn't mind being that close, because I didn't feel like a naughty kid at school who was put in front of the teacher. I hated it because all morning there was a procession of people coming into the unit to have their two-day pre-check. Now we are all the same underneath, but I found it acutely embarrassing that I and the person facing me had to look directly at each other whilst we were both clearly not at our best. I especially felt for some of the older women who had to expose more skin than they would obviously like to have done in front of a complete stranger. This is the way it was, and, rightly or wrongly, it made me almost bolt for the door more quickly than Speedy Gonzales (although I move about as fast as his friend Slowpoke Rodriguez).

As I said, there were to be two drugs given to me during this part of the treatment, but I was booked in from eight in the morning until about half-four in the afternoon. The reason for this was that you don't just walk in, get the good stuff and leg it to your flat to see what happens, like an aging hippy after licking a 'tab'. There are various drips that you are given over the day to ensure that your body copes with this chemotherapy army marching into your arteries like some kind of crusading force. There is saline to keep your fluid levels up and stop your kidneys feeling as if you have just done a two-day session with Keith Moon and Oliver Reid. There are small bags to flush you out, and your fluid intake/output is closely monitored. The fluid intake is a simple procedure, in that you have a sheet on which you list the drinks you have and the volume of each. However, the output requires a slightly more dextrous approach. As you are now hooked up intravenously, you need to unplug the trolley holding your bags of goodies from the wall, then take it and a re-cycled cardboard container in the shape of an oversized kidney (not sure whether that is a generic hospital shape or a pointed reminder that your kidneys are crying out to be considered) into the toilet and pee into the container, measure it and then dispose of it. This was done by placing it in a little cupboard, along with everyone else's, like some strange dumb-waiter where no-one looks forward to pudding.

This is also a good point to mention that some of the side-effects now start to show, and you are very pleased you were advised, because one of the drugs I was given turns your pee redder than the Nile during the Ten Plagues. Imagine the scare and the screams coming from the toilet if I hadn't had that bit of pre-advice. The first chemo drug I was given was the one responsible for my scarlet toilet habits. (No, I don't mean that Rhett Butler should be worried.) The way it is administered is slightly comical, though; well, it seemed so to me. Whilst you are having some saline or such dripped into you, the nurse comes over with the drug in what I can only describe as a huge syringe that would not look out of place being accidentally self-administered by Wile E Coyote. The way it is given is that the nurse sits next to you and slowly injects it over a five-or-so-minute period: not quite the intimate scenario I had pictured in my head, involving myself and a lovely lady dressed in a nurse's uniform, but reality is often slightly more abstract.

The next drug was fed by drip over a two-hour period, and this is when I truly realised that it was all happening: I was really having chemotherapy treatment. I keep saying about the reality thing, but for me this is because, despite being in the appointments and meetings and despite the information going through my ears and being processed by my brain, it all seemed a little abstract to me. Once I was in certain situations, it was all very real, but up until that point it was not unreal - more 'to be confirmed', if that makes sense. I had obviously seen documentaries and dramas where people had such drugs, but it was only when I saw the red bag being hooked up to me that it sank in. (Apparently they are red so that the sunlight does not affect the liquid inside. That must be why gingers have red skin - to protect their blood from boiling, but it can't always work, hence the tantrums. Oh, and I'm allowed: I am said ginger - or was.) It is quite a long day having this treatment, so, despite taking my laptop, mobile, books and some puzzles, I found my mind wandering round the room. The first thing I noticed was a row of strange-looking machines that resembled the big hairdryers you used to see in salons. The only difference was that, instead of a big plastic dome to fit over your head, there was a type of soft cloth cap. I asked one of the nurses what they were for and was informed that they were for ladies having treatment for breast cancer. I immediately started wondering whether anyone was going to expose her chest and was about to say so to the nurse when she added that they were for use on the head, apparently to help with the hair-loss. As I say, wait for all the information.

One of the most annoying things in the ward, as mentioned earlier, was the constant beeping. This was from the pump units we each had that controlled the flow of drugs into our systems. The beeping was to remind the nurses that they had finished whatever course they were on and now needed a new course, a bit like birds in a nest, and just as noisy. In fairness, they weren't too bad when it was just the one, but, when a few ran out at the same time, there was general looking and slightly annoyed glances round the ward. Obviously the nurses were not just standing around chatting: that was only in the afternoons (I jest). The team of nurses and support workers had a very difficult job juggling new patients, pre-checks, drug changes and various other things that cropped up during their shift. However, it is human nature to think you are being ignored if your machine bleeps for more than two minutes: doesn't she realise I have cancer?

Herein lies the problem, though. I joke about being impatient, and to be honest there were things that happened in my chemotherapy sessions that under normal circumstances I should have had a slight issue with, but the simple fact of where you are makes all that impossible, for me at least. On the chemotherapy ward, you can quite easily look to your left or to your right and that person may very well not be there in a very short time, it's that simple. It is not always the case, but it was very prominent in my mind. I was very aware of my own set of circumstances and prospects, and you sometimes hear conversations others have with their visitors that give snippets of information about their case, but on the whole you never really know. All I did know was that one word kept coming to the fore of my mind and would not go away, and that word was 'perspective'. It may not be the right word for all, but for me it changed the whole experience of my cancer treatments in general. Throughout this disease, I have known people who have been diagnosed and died, some in an incredibly short space of time. I have seen the efforts made to help me by family, friends and the NHS as a body. I have questioned my own mortality, morality and general outlook. The overall feeling I have is that I am pretty lucky. My glass is definitely above the halfway-full mark. Some, however, have much shorter and more unpleasant journeys with this awful disease, so for me keeping everything in perspective became quite important.

Well, my first day in treatment came to an end, and I was given a party-bag of more drugs to take home with me. I was just about to waddle off home when one of the nurses came over and made me take some pills that make you urinate. It seemed that my output had not been quite sufficient, and I needed to give some more before they were happy to let me go. Well, I managed to provide sufficient quantity to satisfy Nurse Bossy-Boots and was let out. What she failed to tell me was that the pills would continue to work during the next hour or so - not the best car journey I've ever had. The strange thing for me was that I kind of expected any side-effects to start immediately, but that is not the case, as one nurse advised me. If you are going to have any, they will usually show in the first forty-eight hours. The side-effects I experienced were slightly more pronounced after each session.

That first day I came home and had a bath and an early night, as I was feeling pretty tired. I put that down to the long day I had just been through. The next day, though, I felt about as energetic as a three-toed sloth after taking some downers. I had no energy and crawled back to bed, where I ended up staying for the next five days. I was sleeping eighteen to twenty hours a day, only glancing occasionally at the TV and getting up only to use the bathroom, take pills or make myself something to eat, which, because of either lethargy, lack of appetite or both, was microwave porridge. Apologies to my Scottish family for the use of microwave stuff, but making anything else really wasn't an option. Over that first week I lost about a stone in weight: this cancer is really great for the waistline, but it's definitely not a diet I'd recommend! So after my energy-levels had risen a little on day six, I decided to consult my side-effect book and see whether it warranted a call to the nurses. It did, so I rang in with my temperature at hand to be told not to worry, as it was quite normal! I accepted this and shuffled back to bed. 'Normal' is a word used quite often by various doctors and nurses throughout my treatment. The main thing to remember is that nothing you are going through is completely normal, and there are things that happen that seem downright unnatural. I shan't go into my bowel habits, but what I found was that, if something was happening that I didn't consider normal, I should ask, my thought being that it may not be normal to *me* but that, if a surgeon, doctor or nurse knew about it and had encountered or expected it and said so, I could relax.

The effects I had over the next two cycles of my treatment became worse each time. I did not sleep, as if I had just taken a bite from an apple given to me by an obviously disguised witch in a forest: I mean, what was she thinking? - let alone staying with seven miners in a one-bedroomed cottage! What I did experience was gradually increasing periods of very bad nausea. I can only describe it as the feeling of the room's spinning after several drinks too many combined with the dizziness experienced after getting off a rather extreme rollercoaster. I wasn't vomiting, but that feeling of constantly thinking you are about to is often worse, I think. I was also having some severe balance problems which really annoyed me, as I always hope to have at least a bottle of Bacardi in me before I start using the walls to keep walking in a straight line. These effects lasted about a week after my second cycle and about ten days after my third, but on the whole, if I look at the list I had been given of what I could have suffered, I think I got off more lightly than Mr Simpson (and not the one that goes 'doh!').

On my second cycle of treatment, I noticed a sign on my chair-side table giving details of the unit's Christmas party. (This was now the middle of November.) In a stupid fit of moral responsibility and gratitude, I spoke to one of the nurses organising it and told her that I used to do gigs and perhaps an hour of 'Rat Pack'-style music would go down well. She unfortunately agreed straightaway, so I was duly given the 5pm to 6pm slot at the party. It was supposed to be only between 5pm and 7pm, but, judging by the amount of raffle and auction prizes I saw, I think they may have got away for Boxing Day. Well, the appointed day came, and I turned up and did my hour. I think it went well, bearing in mind the location. Don't worry, no-one was hooked up getting their treatment. In fact people were doing the usual meet-and-greet whilst scoffing sausage-rolls as if there were a food-blockade being imposed the next day. I had several people ask me about other paying gigs for them, but I politely declined, as I had given up that aspect of my singing, although the fact they asked meant I wasn't that bad. For me it was quite a difficult gig for a couple of reasons. Firstly, I cannot remember the last time I had done a gig sober, but, apart from a glass of wine that had Parsons Malt written on the label, I had had nothing. Secondly, over the years, I had worked on and fine-tuned a set list of songs to use, based on my liking them and, more importantly, on whether they suited me. Here, however, I was in a chemotherapy ward, suddenly realising that singing 'My Way,' Sinatra, or 'Return to Me,' Dean Martin, would not exactly suit the moment. 'Sod it,' I thought, 'I'm still singing "That's Life".' I did, and they loved it.

During my day-long visits to the chemotherapy ward for treatment, I noticed that a lot of people would come in and be out again in a couple of hours. 'Jammy buggers,' I thought: strange how cancer patients can get jealous of each other! Again this is down to the scheduled treatment for your personal situation, but I hoped that, if I had to have more chemotherapy after my main operation, it would take the form of one of these flying visits. Like Nixon, and so many before him, I too was very wrong. After your main operation, should you have one, you will more than likely be required to have more chemotherapy or possibly radiotherapy, again dependent on your circumstances. For me it was to be more chemotherapy. Whilst I tried to contain my joy at this thought, I understood the reasoning behind it. Why go through everything you have had to up until now, just to give the bugger even the slightest chance of making a comeback? I really want to say something against the Big Reunion show, but, because I liked it, I'll let you decide.

The fact is that, even though my chemo treatments had not been bad enough to warrant a melancholy song written by Leonard Cohen, it had been bad enough for me to think really long and hard about future treatments.

Now as at this stage I was post-op (no, I wasn't wearing pantyhose, big red lips and calling myself Petunia), I was in the position of knowing that more chemotherapy this time was mainly preventative and of fixed schedule. As I said earlier, there are some patients who were having less intense smaller treatments, and I had hoped desperately that my next cycles would be reduced, but that was not to be. I was to have three cycles exactly the same as previously. The reason I mention thinking long and hard is quite simple but, thank God for me, irrelevant now. If I had been unfortunate enough that the tumour was not operable and I had fallen into the palliative path, I really should have had to consider long and hard whether chemotherapy was a part of any further treatments I wanted to do again. This is something I think we have all heard about and shaken our non-cancerous judgemental heads at, muttering, 'How could you *not* accept treatment?' Well, for me it was a serious consideration. I have been through it, and the truth is that, if I was under palliative treatment and had maybe six months left, I really am pretty sure that I should not want to spend three of them suffering in the ways I had previously. I really do believe that I would rather have taken a drop in my remaining time, refused chemotherapy and gone on a binge bigger than Johnny Holmes' trouser-serpent. The fact is that, if I had had to make that decision, the quality of my remaining time would definitely have outweighed quantity. I do not say this lightly, and I do not consider it easier to say because it is a moot point. I say it because I truly believe that is the decision I should have made, but again I must emphasise that a decision of such magnitude is personal and dependent on many things, such as prognosis, attitude, real awareness of the specific circumstances and responsibility to others. By responsibility I don't mean to your bank-manager in getting your overdraft paid off: I mean to the ones closest to you who have played such an important part in your journey so far and deserve consideration.

Well, I was assigned more chemotherapy as stated and accepted the fact that I was to have another nine weeks of partial misery. Why couldn't Kim Basinger be in my nine weeks? Oh, yeah, half-a-week missing, always coming-up-short me! One of the issues that was taken into consideration for my second round of chemo - ding ding - was that, after my first cycle, there had been the five days of sleeping and not eating, and not in the Kate-Moss-diet way. There was such concern for this and any other issues that may occur post-surgery that I was fitted with a 'feeding jejunostomy' tube during my main op. It is a tube that goes from outside your abdomen, round the navel area (no, not Chatham Dockyard) to your duodenum, and, if you have major issues with eating orally, you can get the required fluids/nutrition into you via the tube. I was also given a feeding-machine and some bags of feed: 'All this could be yours for just £5 here tonight on the Saline of the Century!' (I should point out that there are other ways of non-oral feeding on the market, and I am in no way being sponsored by JejunostomiesЯus!) Again it all gets tailored to the individual case, but the result was I now had a plastic tube sticking out of me, and, as I don't believe they have successfully invented a plastic bullet, I couldn't even say I had got it in battle. What with my ever-expanding scar sites, flaps of skin from weight loss and now this, I really was starting to think I would have more chance of finding Capt Kidd's pirate treasure on Dover seafront than ever getting intimate with a woman again: excellent - a huge improvement in my chances, then. There were many issues with my feeding-tube, and in the end I had to have a replacement put in - but more of that later.

I started my second bout of chemotherapy on Friday 4 April 2014. All my chemo sessions have been on a Friday, which is quite inconsiderate, considering I usually have my mixed nude sky-diving club on a Saturday morning. All was as previously during the treatment, and I went home to be pleasantly surprised that I didn't have the extreme sleeping bouts as before. This happiness was to be very short-lived, as the nausea and lack of appetite hit me like a steam train. The effect on me was that I started losing more weight than Kerry Katona in a good month and felt about as strong as a polo mint. Now these circumstances were exactly why I had a feeding-tube in place, and my concerns would not have been an issue had the dietetic team remembered that they were supposed to have given me the feeding-machine and feeds prior to my chemotherapy treatment: I had the car but no engine or petrol.

By Monday I had some major worries about my deteriorating health but knew I had an appointment with the surgical team in Maidstone on Wednesday, so I just tried to force as much high-calorie food into myself as possible. Now normally a jam doughnut and various other sweet things were a big no-no for me owing to the diabetes, but needs must. On a serious note, regardless of the size you may be, one thing I have learned from medical people over the course of my cancer is that losing weight rapidly is never a good thing. I believe the main reason is that our bodies don't tend to utilise the fat resources we have left waiting for them round our midriffs, like some smorgasbord for cellular feasting. What tends to happen is that the body takes what it needs from places such as around the organs. As I have said many times, I am not medically trained, so this is just what I have gleaned in conversations with doctors and nurses. The upshot is that your kidneys and other vital organs can suffer greatly, even worse than a gentleman's evening where the guest speakers are Louis Walsh and Jedward.

By the Wednesday appointment I was in a pretty poor state: I had lost about a stone and was very weak. The difference this time with the weight-loss was that I still had no appetite and had really bad nausea, unlike the previous time I lost a stone. After that time I seemed to snap out of it and was as ravenous as Yogi Bear after hibernation, and I certainly didn't feel like Boo Boo! It was apparent that the surgeon and nurse I saw shared my concerns, and, as it was late in the day, they began a concerted assault on the dietetic team to make sure I was thoroughly checked on. I finally got hold of the dietician after several phone-calls on Thursday and was told that they would get to see me on Friday and would take things from there. I shall go into my dealings with the NHS in its own chapter, but one important point you need to remember - so I shall mention it here as well - is that they don't always get things right. There are many reasons such as workloads, priorities or what I like to call the H G Wells syndrome: this is where you become the invisible man and simply slip through the cracks. You never need to shout in your dealings with the NHS; you never need to be rude in your dealings with the NHS; but just occasionally you need to listen to your own conscious self and speak up! If you are being silly or worrying over nothing, they will soon tell you and put your mind at rest, but at least you will have asked. They are human, and, much as they always want to, they sometimes don't get things correct all the time. I use 'they' because on many occasions it is the system not an individual that has failed, and it is important to remember this.

So with this in mind I voiced my concern to Ashley, the dietician who called me, that I really didn't feel I could wait another day to start using the feeding-tube, as by now my oral intake was down to zero: a bit like an upset wife. Fortunately for me, Ashley was able to get hold of a lovely nurse, whose name escapes me, and she agreed to come out and bring me some feed and a machine that evening. She did, and she gave me a crash-course on how to use it, and, although the alarm on the machine sounded more times than the boy cried wolf, I felt happier knowing I had halted the decline and was now getting at least some nutrition. Ashley and a nurse came to visit me the next day as agreed, and we had a more detailed meeting, the upshot being that I was right to chase the previous evening and that the equipment should have been in place prior to chemotherapy, as previously agreed. Much sighing, apologising on all parts, and plan-creating later, I had enough feeds to sustain me through any further issues (enough to sustain me through WWIII - so ha, Putin); the knowledge to use the equipment; and most importantly I felt reassured I was being supported.

One slight issue they were concerned about was that I appeared to have developed an infection under my feeding-tube. I pointed out the odious smell emitted by my midriff, whilst swearing I had showered that morning. So I was told that the community nurse would come and see me ASAP to take swabs, and they would speak to my doctor and order me some antibiotics. The feeding-machine itself is only the size of a small radio, and you even get a hip little back-pack to go with it, but it's not something I would recommend taking on a gap year. It is very simple to use, and, even when the errors pop up, they are quite easy to resolve, so I went back to resting up and letting the food drip into me. Unfortunately, this would not be the end of my problems at this time, as by the Monday I was really starting to feel quite unwell and had some real pain under the feeding-tube site. My antibiotics arrived on the Monday – 'I was making love by Wednesday': sorry just wanted to slot that song in! However I really was still pretty weak, sore and tired by this point, but Ashley had said she would come and see me on Tuesday. We had even done the See-you-next-Tuesday joke on parting last, so I knew advice was only a day away. Well, Tuesday came, and Ashley arrived with a nutritional nurse. Within a couple of minutes, it was clear that they wanted me in hospital. I was pretty much against this, as my last couple of hospital stays had issues which are described better in the NHS chapter, but, as by this point I really had run out of any form of argument against going into hospital, I was duly despatched. Well, OK, I thought, I'm overdue a bit of TLC, so let's see how this stay goes. I was in for four days; I talked them into letting me go before the Easter weekend, and I think they thought TLC was the American band that did Waterfalls. Well, I got home and my appetite returned and the infection had cleared up, so all I had to do now was deal with the rest of the chemotherapy symptoms - knowing that, after all this, cycle two was just around the corner.

Cycle two was not bad at all in comparison. It was back to the equivalent cycle first time round, in that there were lots of minor issues but nothing major. One thing I must say at this point is, please do not see what happened to me and think, 'Bugger that,' because, as I keep stating like an unlucky national lottery, it might *not* be you! I must also add that the nurses I dealt with on the chemotherapy ward were absolutely fantastic, both supportive and mentally caring (a word often not applicable to some departments or people). I cannot thank them enough for all the big things they did, like the physical care and all the little things they did, like buying me lunch from the canteen one day in order to make an unpleasant experience a lot more bearable. The only thing that kept me going through the last couple of treatments was the thought that they were the last two and more importantly they were bringing me closer and closer to the final all-clear.

Chapter Nine

The NHS

Of all the chapters in this book I have found this one the most difficult to write, which, considering some of the subject matter in other chapters, gives you an idea of my thinking. It's a bit like going up to a favourite uncle who has just given you a bag of sweets and kicking him where a gentleman should never be kicked. I grew up just knowing that the NHS was there. I wasn't a sickly child or teenager, but I did once come down with glandular fever when I was thirteen or fourteen, which knocked me sideways for a while. My only other dealing with it in my youth was when I was late for school once and decided that a plastic shopping-bag was sufficient to carry my books in whilst I hammered it down the road on my racing-bike. I really should have foreseen this, as I was studying physics at school. Well, a plastic bag suddenly inserted into the wheel spokes at 20-odd mph can have only one outcome: thanks, Mr Newton, you and your bloody laws. Convinced that the paramedic in the resulting ambulance was my geography teacher, I started babbling many excuses as to why my homework was not done; for which I think I blamed my sister. I was despatched to the local A&E, where I proceeded to throw up like the exorcist and was admitted for twenty-four hours' observation for concussion. When you are young you just accept certain things: the sky is blue, water is wet, and parents just don't understand you in the slightest or they would have let you go to the school disco. Didn't they realise you were hoping for some under-coat girl-action after preening like a peacock in a circle of testosterone-fuelled lads giving it their best moves to Madness' 'The Prince'? I never did get to Orange Street.

As you get older, you start to observe and become more aware of things, and the NHS was one of these. I'm not going to get all political, but, as I was growing up, there were many huge political issues, and the NHS was one. All I knew was that I was grateful it existed: it deserved any funding it needed, and nurses were angels in fishnets. I think we all have a romantic vision of how it operates and what it would be like if we ever had to be ensconced in its loving arms, although mine was pretty much based on TV shows such as *Angels*, *Casualty* and of course ... the *Carry On* Films. Recently, as in over the past twenty years or so, there has been much made about shifting funding from ground-floor staff to management teams, which to my mind means a load of non-medical people telling a load of medically trained people that they are doing a great job, but the money is now going on my salary, so we need to cut costs. A bit over-simplified, but these are just my thoughts and opinions.

Anyway, as I first ventured into the system with cancer, my initial dealings were extremely good. I have told you about the procedures, and all in all I cannot be negative, apart from the little food débâcle of the laparoscopy 2013. Sometimes I would come across individuals who clearly saw me on a conveyor belt of symptoms, but the vast majority of people I came across were as I had hoped: caring, understanding and considerate. Unfortunately the fishnets seem to have gone the way of party-seven beer-cans, but there again so has smoking in bed on the ward. As said before, my treatment was split between oncology and surgical, and all my oncology appointments/treatments were to be done at QEQM, Margate, and all surgical procedures at Maidstone. Geographically this was a distance of about fifty miles, but in administrative terms this was about the distance between the earth and the moon. This is when I first realised how the impact of hospitals' being sectioned off into separate trusts affects the patient. The idea behind it is, as very often, good on paper. Since each trust has its area of specialty, the standard of care is higher and the patient gets the best treatment possible. It is probably a lot more complex than that, and this is why I am going to deal only with things that I have come across during my year with cancer and why I am not going to elaborate on the workings and aims of the NHS as a whole.

The first real thing I saw which leaves the people working in the system open to individual interpretation happened when I stayed overnight at the QEQM hospital for my blood-transfusion. When I awoke in the morning, there was obviously an issue with some poor lady in the ward opposite me, and everyone was very busy with this and with handovers etc., so there was no way I was going to start asking where my blood was, like an overindulged nightwalker. Some time later, when things had calmed down a little, there were about five or six care-assistants who decided my ward would be the best place to grab five minutes and have a catch-up. Now whilst I don't mind listening to make-up tips, how Botox is a real consideration and the latest gossip about so-and-so from orthopaedics, Brian the care-assistant really wasn't doing it for me! They waffled on for about five minutes, and the point is that I could quite easily have filmed them on my phone: without the context of the morning they had just had, it could easily have been made to look as if they were just stood around all day doing nothing, when the truth was quite the opposite. So this event made me a little more protective of the staff I was dealing with and a little more dubious of some so-called exposé documentaries. All was well with things, apart from really minor gripes, which are probably just me being picky - like the fact that many of the appointments I had involved people taking time off work to drive me quite some distance, only to discover it was just a catch-up chat to see how I was doing: something I felt could easily have been done on the phone. This was usually at Maidstone hospital. Another irk was that the appointments always ran about an hour behind and usually involved me sitting in a waiting-room full of people sniffing and sneezing, which was not really great if I was in the middle of a chemo cycle.

The major issue I had was really with just one hospital, and it happened mainly on one ward, but the general gripes I had were to do with this hospital in general. Going back to the idea of trusts, there are many problems that I encountered which I am sure would not have happened in the good old days when the NHS was one big happy family. To me it appears that a trust is an independent thing:

Yes, it answers to the same set of rules in general, but there is flexibility in its approach, and therefore it can deviate quite widely from how a different trust will operate. It seems that the trust is steered by its board of management to achieve their particular aims. Now this could mean that they become a centre of excellence for a particular type of disease etc. and therefore they receive more funding and they progress further, which can only benefit the patient suffering from that particular condition, but it just seems to me that it only separates the general population of patients from them. The other issue is that the particular management-style filters all the way down to every department, and this can lead to complacency, lethargy or downright disenchantment. The types of issues this caused me were simple things, such as the fact that certain trusts cannot automatically see your latest test results or planned treatments because the other trust has control of it. I still find it astonishing in today's technological daily workings that the NHS still does not have every patient's details available on computer for all hospitals to see; they still use pen and paper.

Now I am not talking about the security of personal information and its sale to outside bodies, much hyped in the media. I merely cannot understand why all records are not available to all departments/hospitals/trusts at the same time. This isn't Bletchley Park we are talking about, and it's not a need-to-know operating basis. I really think that, if Maidstone is going to operate on my feeding-tube, Margate should know I have one fitted without having to wait three days for my file to arrive from storage. It's the equivalent to a family of four all trying to use the kitchen, each to cook a quarter of the family dinner without the other members knowing what they are doing. Believe me, Shirley, your gravy isn't that good. Now this to me can lead to problems as small as having to explain on every visit/appointment that I have been called Paul all my life and, if it's not toooo inconvenient, it would be nice if you could call me Paul as well. It would be good to be in a position where you the patient are not liaising between separate trusts and hospitals to try to get results of your latest scan or to arrange the next part of your treatment - and I am not making this part up.

To me the NHS is one body with one aim, and that is the care of the good people of this country regardless of financial standing. The same care and treatment should be available anywhere. We have all heard of certain treatments being a postcode lottery. Well, that way of working goes from treatments all the way down to the basic operating procedures of these trusts and unfortunately the outcome is

not always the best for the patient or the NHS itself. As we know, the road to hell is paved with good intentions.

What I am going to do now is mention some of the problems I encountered. I do not do this to gripe, moan or cause any issues for the NHS. After all, there's a pretty good chance I would not be here if the NHS didn't exist or had not progressed and developed significantly in the past few decades since my great bike smash of '79. The reason I list them is that this is what I experienced in my year with cancer. If it makes someone more aware and therefore able to avoid the same problems in their treatment, great; if it makes anyone in the system want to look into it in a positive way to try to fix it, even better. I guess the first time you encounter a problem in your treatment-plan, it is a bit of a surprise. Sort of like when Jessica Rabbit first appears on screen: it's a cartoon, why am I staring at her boobs? As mentioned before, the first time I felt a little miffed with my treatment was after my laparoscopy, when I was in the recovery-ward. It wasn't just the food issue: it was the fact that I was in a bay of eight beds, and I was the only person for the first couple of hours, and apart from my observations being taken (without any form of conversation) every hour I was left alone. If the staff are busy, you can understand, but when they are quite obviously not, you wonder whether your deodorant is really working. This made me feel, as it would on many occasions to come, that the best thing I could do was get out of there quickly.

The next problem I encountered was more of confusion over my planned operation. The first issue was that, in the three appointments I had at Maidstone to discuss the operation with the surgical team, I never saw the same person twice, and, although the general gist of what was to be done was the same, they all had different opinions of the peripheries. The main point, though, was that the operation would be an open-chest job. Since an oesophagectomy is apparently one of the most invasive and serious operations they perform in this country, taking it all in is quite a scary thing to do: worse even than finding out that the girl walking down the aisle to you was once a lorry driver from Scunthorpe called Bob! One of the most important considerations for this operation is that it will not be done if the surgical team feel that they cannot get all the cancer during surgery. The surgical team told me that this was the only way the operation could be performed, so I accepted that. It was only when I had discovered that the chemotherapy sessions had indeed worked and that the tumour had become detached enough so that it was indeed operable, that I went to see the surgeon for confirmation of this and was informed that they would no longer be doing the operation at Maidstone and that I was being transferred to Guy's and St Thomas'. That in itself was a surprise, but the bigger surprise was that, when I went to London to discuss my operation with the surgeon there, I was told that it may well be performed laparoscopically, which was never mentioned by Maidstone. I later found out there was a reason why Maidstone would not do the operation any way other than by open surgery and why I was therefore being transferred to London. The alleged reason was that there had been some deaths during this laparoscopic type of surgery over the previous year or so, and, although there was apparently no negligence found, it was alleged that procedures could have been tighter and that things could have been done differently. I believe that one of the deceased patients' families was in the process of taking legal action, so all operations of this type were suspended at Maidstone.

One problem that did quite upset me and shows the issues you can have when dealing with the different hospitals was finding out whether my first three cycles of chemotherapy had indeed been successful. My last session of the three was in the first week of November 2013. I was aware that no operations can take place for at least six weeks after chemotherapy, and this is because the one thing in your body that chemo really takes its toll on is your bone marrow. So I knew that nothing could happen until December, but the sense of urgency in finding out whether the chemo had worked was quite important to me, as I'm sure you can understand. The way things had been described to me was that I was to have a CT scan post-chemo, and then my oncologist would discuss the results with me. The tumour would be either operable or not from the oncological point of view. This assessment would then be passed to the surgical team, and they would either confirm the prognosis or not. As I said, my last chemotherapy treatment was on 6 November, and technically part of the treatment was a course of tablets for three weeks. I therefore felt I couldn't chase anything until that had been completed. Again I was back in the waiting game, this time to find out whether I was indeed able to have the operation or was again looking at that word palliative. This was quite a stressful time for me, as you can probably imagine, but the fact that the three-week period post-chemo came and went and I still had not heard from anyone started to concern me. I then decided a gentle nudge to the relevant parties was in order: by 'gentle nudge' I mean sledgehammer and by 'parties' I mean walnuts.

One thing that added to my frustration was that I received an appointment to see my oncologist when I hadn't even had an appointment for a scan! Eventually, after several phone calls to various departments (remember I am dealing with two different trusts), I managed to get a CT scan booked for Sunday 8 December and rearrange my appointment with my oncologist for the Monday, having been reassured by the CT department that the scan images would be available for Dr Waters to see. Fortunately, the scan and appointment came under the same trust. However, even then the write-up would not be available until a few days later. I also managed to ensure I had an appointment with the surgical team for the 11th, so I was quite pleased with my efforts to get the ball rolling again: a bit like Status Quo on reunion-tour number fifty-six. As mentioned, my oncologist gave me the fantastic news that he considered it operable, and the surgeon I saw at Maidstone agreed, but it was then I found out that my surgery had been transferred to St Thomas' in London. The nurse at the surgical consultation stated that she would fax all the details to London that evening, and I should receive an appointment there within the week and definitely before Christmas. This was all a big relief to me, and it meant that I had a fighting chance and would be able to go and see my family in Glasgow for Christmas, as I had hoped to do.

By the week after, however, when I had still not heard from St Thomas', I again took the bull by the horns and chased the trust up. After some chasing, I was given an appointment for the 18th only for the specialist nurse to call me the next day and tell me it would have to be rearranged, as the secretary arranging it had 'lots of appointments for various clinics to schedule, and she had got this one wrong'. She also stated that they had never received any faxed information about my transfer. Fortunately, it was rearranged for the day after, but being talked down to by this new specialist nurse did not bode well for me and my new relationship with a London hospital. As it happens, I was correct about the new specialist nurse, as, during this appointment and the couple of dealings I had with her post-surgery, she gave the distinct impression that the whole situation was about her and what she does, so I must take this opportunity to apologise to her if my cancer got in the way of her plans.

Well, I met the surgeon, who informed me about the operation. To be honest, his appearance took me a little by surprise. During my chat with Specialist Nurse What-Would-They-Do-Without-Me - probably have to book some new dramas - she had a couple of doctors etc. popping in to discuss things. 'They just can't cope without me,' she boasted. One such interruption was by a middle-aged chap in a white boiler-suit that I assumed (that word again) was doing some general maintenance in the corridor that needed the approval of Specialist Nurse 'A'-Team-Hannibal-Smith. He disappeared only to reappear a few minutes later and introduce himself as Professor Mason who would be doing my surgery. This relaxed me, and the good professor talked me through all the details, such as how many they had done and the fact that this operation was previously always done there prior to Maidstone taking over. Most importantly, he seemed to take the time to ensure I understood everything, which put me greatly at ease, considering the operation I was about to have. At the time, I just thought he was trying to reassure me over the op, but with hindsight I believe the issues facing Maidstone and the transfer of these operations was foremost in his mind. I asked when the op might take place, and, checking his calendar and confirming that I should be beyond the six-week bone-marrow concerns, he said, 'Tuesday 7 January' - at which point Nurse Hannibal

Smith tried to convince him that would be too soon. To my relief, he told her that date would be fine, and I smiled inwardly, not just because of this now-confirmed date but because I had the great pleasure of seeing Hannibal Smith return to her computer-screen with a face that looked as if someone had come into her house on Christmas morning and pee'd on all her presents: glorious! I then had all my pre-operation checks and headed home, knowing that I had a date and could enjoy Christmas. All things considered, I was very very happy.

One other thing that quite upset me was that, during this time, I was emotionally really starting to feel the pressure again, and, although it is not in my nature to go for counselling-type things, I did feel that it might be something I should look into, as I really was having a period of not coping very well with the added stress of trying to sort everything. This is a subject mentioned elsewhere, but this part fits with this chapter. I made contact with the oncology team and was informed that the counselling nurse would be in contact with me. At this stage I was still going to work, and I duly received a call from said nurse. I shall quote you the call and allow you to draw your own conclusions, bearing in mind I am pretty reluctant to open up, being a full-blown macho man: OK, a repressed idiot, and I was surrounded by work colleagues when I received the call.

Nurse: 'Hi, is that Robert?'

'It's Paul, but yes.'

'Well, I need to speak to Robert.'

'I am Robert, but I'm always called Paul: sorry, it's a family heirloom thing.' Nervous chuckle: yes, this again!

'So you are Robert?' – a slightly agitated tone.

'Yes, but it's Paul I prefer.'

'So, Robert, I understand you want some counselling.'

By this time my work colleagues are picking up on the conversation.

'I'm not sure.'

'OK, well, if you change your mind, give us a ring.' She then hangs up.

I had my operation as detailed in its own chapter, but one thing I shall mention here is that you have to book into the hospital the day prior to surgery. I therefore arrived on Monday 6th and was put on to a ward. It was that evening that I met the surgeon to discuss the operation, and to my slight alarm it was not Professor Mason: it was Mr James Gossage. Now the fact that this chap was a lot younger made me slightly nervous but less than the fact that this was described to me as a major operation, and I had only just managed to put the jitters away, and here was someone I had never met before telling me how they were going to slice me and remove bits of me like some late-night kebab-vendor. Suffice it to say I was more nervous than a 70s' DJ from *Top of the Pops* when there's a knock on the front door! All I can add to this is that continuity would have been much appreciated, but the surgeon himself, Mr Gossage, did an excellent job on the surgery, which even medical staff comment on to this day. At every post-op meeting I had with him, he exuded a knowledgeable, professional, understanding and caring attitude. To my way of thinking, I really did have the best man for the job, although I still think he slipped with the scalpel and added eight inches to my scar by accident (joke, sir, joke!).

One of the things that caused me the most problems over the course of my treatment was my jejunal feeding-tube. This is a tube that was surgically put in place during my time at St Thomas' and is to enable you to feed via specialist feed-bags (sound like a budgerigar), should you be unable to eat orally for whatever reason. The simple fact that you have a tube hanging out of you is problematic enough, but the issues began a month or so after surgery. The tube goes into me about an inch above my navel and about three inches to the left of it. It is held in place by a triangular flange which on my first tube (I see you know where this is going) was about an inch below the entry site of the tube, and it was held in place by two stitches. I should have foreseen the issues when I had to have one of the stitches redone on my appointment back at St Thomas' two weeks after my discharge. The problem I had was that the stitches kept falling out. It seemed to me that the stitch would be inserted, a scab would form round the area and then fall off taking the stitch with it. Hang on! Perhaps I have discovered some weird form of perpetual motion. I was given the contact-details of something called the HEN team (Home Enteral Nutrition), who would be assisting me with nutrition and other issues relating to my feeding etc. whilst I had this tube in place. They were supposed to contact me on my discharge from hospital, but, surprisingly enough, they were never passed my details, and I got in touch with them only after a call to my GP's surgery to seek advice after a stitch came out the first time at home. After some digging by my GP's receptionist, my details were passed to them. They gave me a letter to take to any A&E department if the stitches came out, so that I could be 'seen quickly and have the site re-stitched with the minimum of fuss', as they said this was my only option.

Well, I think you may guess whether that worked! At first I felt that one stitch would suffice, but eventually the other decided to give up the ghost and join its fallen comrade, so, after a quick call to my friends Jo and Mof, I went to Ashford A&E. I had already called the department to try and pre-advise them so as to minimise my wait. Now don't get me wrong: I do not mind waiting my turn in an A&E department, but when you are surrounded by people who are there mainly because they cannot get an appointment with their GP or cannot be bothered to check alternative options available to them (sometimes just down the corridor, such as walk-in clinics), and all this whilst suffering from the lovely effects of chemotherapy, you obviously try and minimise your wait if possible. This first time was not bad at all, and eventually I had a lovely young doctor asking me to lie down and lift my top; and, yes, she was female! As I was re-stitched and on my way home in less than two hours, I was very happy. The only event of note took place whilst myself, Jo and Mof waited in my cubicle for the doctor: the woman who was in the cubicle next to us decided to let off an almighty gust of wind. Not again, I thought, I can't do Monty Python at the moment.

My happiness, however, was short-lived, as my two new stitches decided they didn't like me, and both committed stitchicide within three days. One went the next day, and his mate pined so much he went on the Friday. So another call to Jo, and back to Ashford A&E I went. This time was quite different, unfortunately, as none of my pre-arrival planning paid any dividends, and, after a couple of hours in the audience of a Jeremy Kyle episode, I was triaged and then went back to waiting. Eventually, just as I was about to hit their four-hour limit for dealing with me, I was taken to another section and examined further. The upshot was that the doctors didn't want just to re-stitch the site, despite my waiving my white please-re-stitch-him letter in the air with the fervour of a Frenchman in 1940. Their concern, and I have to accept their decision, was that the tube might have moved out of its correct position in my duodenum and therefore the tube would be no use when, and if, required. I tried to point out to them that at several times previously the tube had come out of the site by as much as three inches, but this only seemed to make them more determined. The outcome was that I was moved round to a CDU (Clinical Decision Unit) to await a surgeon to look into the matter.

Since I was promised by the nurse as I left the A&E area that a surgeon would see me within the next fifteen minutes, I, Jo and Mof, who had joined us from work, bless him (well, nothing was waiting at home for him), waited for the surgeon to arrive like the cavalry. After a couple of hours, I decided to chase this and was told by the ward-receptionist it would be another couple of hours. I also had the benefit of the fact that Jo knew one of the nurses on the ward, and they made it quite clear that I should be lucky if I saw anyone before the next day. I then did something I am not proud of but still feel it was the correct decision: I discharged myself. I did not take this decision lightly, but after spending more time in hospital recently than Steve McQueen's character spent in the cooler, I decided to do likewise and make my own great escape. To be fair to the ward, they were all very nice and understanding, and some even agreed with me, which made my decision a little easier.

However, please be warned that if you ever do decide to make this decision, you must base it on knowledge of your own situation. I, for example, knew I would not be seen till the next morning; that I was in no immediate danger; being at home would be easier for me with my meds etc. and I would not be taking up a hospital-bed unnecessarily. You must ensure that your decision does not compromise your treatment. I did not, however, get away scot-free, as, when I was leaving, I bumped into the doctor who had made the decision not to re-stitch, and after a chat he seemed disappointed (in the outcome rather than with my decision) and insisted that I receive a new dressing to the tube-site before leaving. I told him I would be fine and I had plenty of dressings at home, but he insisted and called a nurse from A&E over and asked her to do this. I'm unsure who was more embarrassed, myself or the doctor when she returned and stated, 'Well, if he's leaving I'm sure he doesn't mind doing it himself,' whilst shoving some dressings into my hand, which was unfortunately protecting the tube-site at the time. I decided to leave before I exploded like a 1000lb WWII bomb that's just been disturbed from its slumber by a JCB and left the doctor with a stunned expression on his face to deal with her. Hell hath no fury like a scorned A&E nurse.

Well, I knew that I should have to get the tube sorted, but, after the eight or so hours at Ashford, I was just happy to get home. The next day, whilst I was debating my next move to resolve this, I did my normal routine of flushing the tube (it needs to be rinsed through with some sterile water every day) and changing the dressing over the site. Unfortunately, as I took the dressing off, I noticed that the tube had come out of the entry-site by quite some distance, and, as I carefully tried to pull away the rest of the dressing, the remainder of the tube plopped on to my stomach like a new-born, but without the screaming. OK, I may have screamed a little. I knew that this was quite bad, and there was limited time before the wound-site would start to heal itself, so I made contact with the HEN team and, surprise, surprise, was instructed to go to A&E.

This time, however, I decided to give Margate a go, and the HEN team said they would pre-advise them of my situation. I arrived at the QEQM and was taken through to my cubicle pretty quickly, but the problem was that, because the tube had come out, it again required a surgical intervention, and no one at Margate or Ashford - glad I hadn't waited! - was able to re-insert the tube. It had to be done either at Maidstone or back at St Thomas'. Then came the question I was to be asked many times in the coming weeks: Why do you want the tube put back? I was quite stunned by this, as it was a bit like asking someone who has been given some prescription tablets why they then wished to take them. The fact is, I didn't want it in. It was causing me more problems than any other of my treatments, but, as far as I was aware, St Thomas' wanted it in place, and so did my dietetic team. The reason was that it was a precaution in case it was needed when I was recovering from a major operation and the eating issues I had already had previously during my chemotherapy cycles returned. I told the surgeon at QEQM this, and he just said he would speak to St Thomas' again.

The upshot was that, after more phone-calls than the White House received after Ms Lewinski blabbed, the team at QEQM would put in place an alternative tube, in this case a catheter, to keep the site open until I could have a replacement tube inserted by either Maidstone or London. This was a fun procedure, as the surgeon had to try to feed the new tube through the now-empty route of the old tube, but unfortunately the only way he could establish whether he had taken a wrong turning, so to speak, was if I yelped in pain like a dog whose foot you have just stood on. Eventually he conceded that the new tube was not going to go back in, so they just left it as far as they could under the skin in order to keep the wound open to aid the replacement. That done, I was allowed to go home. I must add here, though, that it was not all doom and gloom, as, when the sister in charge of the A&E department realised I had been at Ashford all day previously, at QEQM for a good six hours and then had the joy of getting home on public transport, she took me to one side and told me I had been through enough and the department would get me a taxi home. I didn't get her name, but bless you for that.

The next problem I had (really sorry, but a few more to get through: perhaps have a break and a nice chocolate biscuit to lift your spirits) was that, a couple of days after the temporary tube had been put in, I noticed some blood coming back up it and it was even more sore than the site normally is, to the point I had taken some morphine tablets to ease the pain. Again I reported this to the HEN team and my specialist nurse-department, and the outcome was that, after consulting with St Thomas', they suggested that my best option was to go to the A&E at St Thomas' where they would be able to assess it and look at the option of fitting a replacement. There were a couple of points that concerned me with this suggestion. It was now about 4pm on a Friday evening, and my only way of getting to London was by train, with a painful wound-site, let alone post-op fatigue and other physical problems. This would have put me in a central London hospital's A&E department at about 7pm on a Friday evening. Despite the suggestion to go up to their A&E, I should not be given any consideration of my situation, and there was no plan in place for me to be dealt with, let alone for a replacement tube to be put in: it was a case of let's-look-and-see. After due consideration, I did what Ms Lewinski should have done and declined. No surprise there, and no surprise to find that the suggestion had come from ... Specialist Nurse Hannibal! I then had a chat with the HEN team, and it was agreed that the blood was probably residual from when they tried to insert the catheter and that, as I had some pain relief, I should just monitor the situation. They would try and get me an appointment to have the tube replaced as soon as possible.

I was given an appointment to see the surgical team a week or so later, and we discussed a procedure I was going to have called a pyloric dilatation, which is a procedure to widen the tube, leaving my stomach to help me with some eating issues I was having. The surgeon then turned his attention to my feeding-tube issues and asked the question, 'So why do you want it put back in?' At this point I tried my best to suppress an outburst of frustration, but I'm pretty sure even he spotted the steam escaping from my ears (the only thing missing was a can of spinach). Well, it was decided that I would have the tube replaced as soon as possible, so off I went to await the appointments. After several days I still had not received any appointment-dates, and it was getting very close to my first cycle of chemotherapy, and I was obviously quite keen that nothing should delay that. I chased a few departments and explained that the tube was not in place, and the whole point of my having it, as far as I was aware, was as a precaution, especially for during my chemotherapy cycles.

The week of my chemotherapy arrived, and I still had not had any appointments, so I chased again, and a day or so later I received several appointments, for the tube reinsertion, the pre-op checks for the dilatation and the date for the dilatation itself. The tube-reinsertion was scheduled for the Monday after my first treatment of chemotherapy, despite my best efforts, and the pyloric dilatation would be moved from its planned date to the same day. This meant that, when I went for my pre-chemo checks on the Wednesday, the nurse was very worried that the tube would not be in place. She spoke to my oncologist, and my chemotherapy treatment was postponed till the following week. The only thing that stopped my slumping into a pit deeper than Gordon Brown's pockets on budget day was one of the specialist nurses at the oncology department called Sue Levitt. This is the nurse who had discussed my original plan for treatments after my initial diagnosis. Sue took the time to have a talk with me and gave me a much-needed sympathetic listening ear and an emotional shoulder to lean on. More about Sue in a while, but after a chat I accepted there was nothing I could do, and, despite my efforts, things were as they were.

I arrived at Maidstone hospital on the Monday afternoon to have my two procedures done. Another issue is that if you are not scheduled for first thing, they tell you to stay at home and wait for a phone-call, which is fine if you live round the corner and have someone to take you to the hospital. Having neither, I asked the nice booking-lady what I should do, and we decided the best thing was for me to get there at midday and take it from there: lovely! I went under the knife at about half-four and, when I awoke in the recovery-room, I was immediately overtaken by such pain as I can honestly say I had never experienced previously. It felt as if I were John Hurt and that bloody alien was trying to burst out of my abdomen. After about twenty minutes of people scurrying round me, they finally gave me something that got it under control. I then spent a good fifteen minutes apologising to all and sundry for my loud screams and general outbursts of agony. Most were fantastic, and I was fortunate in that, as I was the last op of the day and the only patient in the recovery-room, no-one else had to suffer my outburst.

Once I was calm, it was decided that I should be admitted to a ward. So I was wheeled round to the appointed ward, hooked up to a pain-relief machine and got some much-needed rest. I know that lots of the things I mention in this section may appear to be trivial matters, and I really hope I don't come across as a moany bugger, but, as I stated at the start, this book is about my experience, and there are many positives. The reality is, however, that these things happened to me, so need to be included if I am to be 100% honest about my year. I say this because one of the biggest problems I have had was specifically to do with my experience on this particular ward at Maidstone hospital. My first inkling that there was an issue was the next morning, when the surgeon who had performed my procedures – again, not the one who had the discussion with me - came to see me. We went through a couple of things about the dilatation procedure etc., but what sort of stopped me in my tracks was when the surgeon looked me in the eyes and said, 'I just can't understand why you were in so much pain!' At first I was unsure whether he was metaphorically scratching his head wondering what had caused it, but then I realised by his expression of questioning that he genuinely must have thought I was making it up or exaggerating.

Since this procedure, I have learned that, apart from the surgeon's making a separate incision parallel to the entry site for some reason which then turned to scar tissue, I was advised that this is quite a painful operation, but this time I did not have the benefit of an epidural - which I did under my main operation. One thing I did think in hindsight was that perhaps this surgical department was now a little more defensive after certain events, but I shall never really know. However, I just found it quite uncomfortable to be practically accused, by a surgeon no less, of feigning pain.

I spent the next two days pumping myself full of more morphine than is probably legal or advisable, which either meant I really was suffering or psychosomatically the pain-fairies in my brain were continuing to make me pretend something was there that wasn't - a bit like any politician's manifesto. My real issue, though, happened on the Wednesday morning, when I crossed the path of someone whom I shall name, quite aptly, Nurse Ratchet. The thing with the self-administered pain-relief is that it can be quite difficult sometimes to find the balance between keeping the pain under control and turning yourself into a zombie, constantly on the verge of sleep and the outskirts of reality: a bit like Norwich. (Don't rise in arms, you Norfolk folk. I lived there for a couple of years and loved it: with a women-to-men ratio of 7:1, I couldn't fail!)

There obviously comes a point where the pain-management team encourage you to come off the machine and go on to alternative relief, which is administered as needed by the nurses. This obviously makes sense, otherwise you would become convinced that any reduction in your pain-meds would instantly result in your lapsing into a state of sheer panic. It should never happen, and the simple fact is that, with lots of these issues and treatments, sometimes you need to lower the defences, be they pain-meds or other meds, to see whether the underlying issue is still there. So it was agreed that I should be unhooked from the good stuff in the presence of Nurse R, and that I should be monitored to see how things were.

Before I go into what happened next, I should advise you of one thing. By this time I have gained, and you will too, a fair bit of knowledge of my specific case, and I am not the type of person who will let an obvious mistake be discussed in front of me without mentioning it. This was something as trivial as what meds I had taken during the previous night, but I knew as soon as the words had left my mouth that I had made a huge mistake by how Ms Ratchet stared at me in a way usually only reserved for the real talentless fantasists on reality TV shows. So there I was, watching my pain-relief machine being taken from me and pining after it like an overprotective dad as his eldest goes off to university. The reality was that, although my pain-level had reduced significantly, I was still in a lot of discomfort and looking forward to a little assistance. This was about 8.30am, and I was rather stunned as Ms Ratchet made a conscious effort to visit every bed on the ward apart from mine to enquire how the occupants were, like some over-indulged petulant teenager in the playground who has the only set of jacks and makes sure everyone knows it. I started to realise the error I had made, despite my requesting via the one and only nursing assistant who came near my bed - which I shall now call the Falklands owing to its exclusion-zone. It was on the 12.30 medication round that Nurse Hand-That-Rocks-The-Cradle came reluctantly into my bed-area. 'Well, Robert, I take it you want some meds!' the 'Robert' being deliberately emphasised despite her having written 'prefers Paul' on the whiteboard above my bed! I pointed out that I was and had been in some quite considerable discomfort all morning, at which she just smiled and advised me that I 'should have asked'. I pointed out that I had and was advised by her, with a grin the Cheshire Cat would have envied, that 'they had been very busy'.

Feeling at this point as vulnerable as a seal sitting on an iceberg while several orcas circled, I decided my best tack was to take the pain-meds she finally got me and try and become the invisible man as far as she was concerned - and also as far as her colleagues, whose attitude to me turned more quickly than Thomas the Tank Engine on a turntable and a promise from Sasha the shed tractor, were concerned. I can only assume - again that Ms R had told a tale of woe about horrid old me. The upshot was that I now felt about as welcome as Herr Schmidt in the Hare & Hounds outside Biggin Hill in 1940. It was during the night-shift, when petty acts with knowing smiles were committed, that I decided that, regardless of the doctor's visit in the morning, I should be leaving this hospital the next day by hook or by crook. Despite having quite an uncomfortable night in terms of pain, I was still adamant the next morning that I should not remain in this hospital, especially when Nurse Ratchet walked in to take over the next day's shift as well. So that's what it looks like when the cat gets the cream, I thought, as she flounced round the ward like a cross between Florence Nightingale and Eva Braun.

Two things happened that morning that lifted my spirits immensely. The first was when the doctor came to see me and, after a chat, agreed that probably the best place for me to be was at home. There was no discussion with Ms R: he based his judgement on my recovery after the surgery. The second was that something must have been said to the aforementioned nurse, since she began the day as if yesterday had not happened and was so overly anxious to fuss over me that I worried she was secretly plotting to close the curtains around me and instruct me personally on the best forms of euthanasia. I don't know whether her change was due to an overnight attack of remorse, or perhaps she had received some advice from a colleague telling her to be a bit more cautious in her one-woman crusade for personal respect and glory. I think she made a mess in her pants thinking about the consequences of her actions if it were ever taken further. Either way, I liked this new Ratchet less than the previous one. The forced attitude and smile made her look like some demonic doll which I'm guessing wouldn't make the ToysЯUs Christmas top-ten list.

Eventually, later that afternoon, I managed to get out of there and felt happier than Hugh Heffner on a bunny-choosing day to be safely back in my flat. Over the next few days I started to wonder whether the events on that ward had happened or whether I had misinterpreted the situation. Eventually I convinced myself that it was probably me being silly and that I was blowing things up in my own mind. It was only after I went for my next chemotherapy treatment and one of the nurses asked me how I had got on at Maidstone that I talked through what had happened with someone in the job. To say they were shocked and disgusted was a little bit of an understatement. They also told me of their own personal dealings with this hospital, which made me feel I wasn't going mad or turning into Victor Meldrew.

I had my first chemotherapy session of this set of treatments on 4 April, and at least I now had the feeding-tube in place. However, what I did not have, despite the HEN team dietician who visited me saying I should have, was the equipment to enable me to use it. 'Not to worry,' I thought. How wrong I was! The reason for the feeding-tube's being in place, according to St Thomas' and my dietetic team, was simply as a precaution based on my chemo-sessions in 2013, as I have mentioned. So I went into my new set of chemo expecting pretty much the same as the previous year's. Unfortunately this was not to be the case. After my first session I did not have the expected days of sleep. I waited. Instead I felt extreme nausea and lack of appetite more associated with the later cycles. The upshot of this was that I stopped eating and lost about a stone in the first five days. I also developed an infection under the feeding-site, as previously mentioned. I discuss all this in the chemotherapy section, but the reason I include it here is to do with the hospital stay. After it was decided that I needed to be admitted, I spoke to Sue Levitt, and she broke the news to me that I should unfortunately need to go to Maidstone Hospital again. She was very aware of the previous problems and was very supportive, but because the surgery had been done there it had to come under their surgical department. She did advise me, though, that I could request at the hospital not to go on to the ward I had had issues with, which made me a little worried, as the last thing I wanted to do was turn up at someone's hospital and start slating one of their sections.

The plan was that, as a surgeon had agreed to see me the next morning, I was to go to A&E, who were expecting me, and they would keep me until the surgeon visited and decided the best way forward. I got to the A&E department, and they were great, very kind and supportive. I also had a chat with a lovely nurse and asked about not going on to ward Stalag-Luft Ratchet, and she was very understanding and took note, which was a great relief. It was about 11pm, however, that they informed me that I should be getting transferred to the Pembury Hospital at Tunbridge, as all surgical cases were dealt with there. I did point out that the plan had been for me to stay where I was, and the surgeon had added me to his list to be seen in the morning, but they convinced me that Pembury was where I should be dealt with. So I was moved the ten miles or so and placed in the ward that looked after pre-surgical cases. Having to explain everything from diagnosis to the present situation to an on-call doctor whilst in quite a bit of discomfort after a draughty half hour ambulance ride, was, to say the least, not my favourite part, but we got there, and, more importantly, they put me on some pain-relief and IV antibiotics to get a start on the infection.

In the morning I met the ward-sister who, I have to say, was an infectiously good-natured lovely lady, and this was a Godsend, as she informed me that they had indeed made an error in transferring me, as the aforementioned surgeon had gone to find me at Maidstone and was quite miffed at finding an empty bed. So the plan was for me to get back to Maidstone. Again I took the opportunity to voice my request not to go on *that* ward, and again she was very sympathetic and said she would do what she could. As the morning passed by and the smells of food from neighbouring bays drifted past my nose, even the discomfort I was in couldn't stop me looking at my 'Nil by mouth'-sign and thinking I am definitely going to ignore the 'please do not feed' signs next time I visit the zoo. It definitely appeared that the antibiotics were working, and my appetite was returning, which I should have thought would be something the department would be pleased about, but apparently not. Late in the morning, I asked where we were with my transfer and was advised that, because I was now 'in the system', they would transfer me only when they could find me a suitable bed back at Maidstone. This meant that, because I was not on an A&E list, I was beyond the four-hour requirement to sort me, so not a great priority. Eventually, at 11pm that evening, I was taken back to Maidstone - to the very ward I had pleaded not to go to - and the very first person I saw was Nurse Ratchet! If I had been able to get off my trolley, I should have beaten Mr Bolt without question. I was put on to a bay and to my great relief soon discovered the playground bully was on a different one. However, it appeared that my name was engraved on their collective memory, so things didn't bode well. Ironic that I should mention my name, as, for the first twelve hours, the name above my bed stayed as the previous patient's until the next morning, when the handover nurse pointed it out to the day-shift, whereon it was quickly changed to Mr Robert Ping! My first real inkling that things were no different came during that first night. As it had been a private company that had transferred me, they were uninsured to have my drip running whilst they moved me, so it was duly turned off and re-hung on a stand by a nurse on my admission to my favourite ward. (I'd like to see Julie Andrews put a positive spin on this ward.) The only problem was that it was a couple of hours later when I eventually saw another nurse and asked for the re-hung drip to be reconnected to me!!! I don't usually get much sleep when I am in discomfort, so when the night shift came to check on my drip, if the alarm sounded, I was hopeful of some form of human contact, but sadly they seemed to think a quick look at the drip and a cancellation of the alarm was sufficient. Oh, to be a social pariah!

The next day I was unable to see the surgeon who had agreed to take me under his care, as he was not at Maidstone, but some of his team came, and so began a war of attrition based on my knowledge of the immediate situation and their protocols. The problem was that I was starting to improve - down to the antibiotics - and my appetite had started to improve, so I naturally thought the best thing for me would be to eat. Even the nurse on duty the next day agreed. So there I was, looking forward to some lunch when the surgical team came in and stated they wanted me kept nil by mouth until they had established the exact extent of the problem. If I was lucky, they might allow me a soft diet the next day. I tried to explain my thinking, in that the two-day delay in seeing them had resulted in the antibiotics' working and the priority surely (it is, but don't call me Shirley ... love that film) was for me to start eating again; but alas, their protocols dictated otherwise. This was also the case for the dietician who saw me in rather a deflated and depressed mood – me, not her. Her protocols dictated that I start using the feeding-tube slowly to ensure it was working, then gradually to increase the dose and then to return me to oral nutrition. My thinking was that we needed to establish whether the tube was indeed working now that the infection was clearing up. (That reminds me to thank the lovely nurse on my arrival at that ward who looked at my tube-site, after my explaining what was going on, and declared in a more sarcastic manner than Frankie Boyle, 'Well, it doesn't look infected to me, looks fine,' whilst giving me her best you're-a-hypochondriac stare and then flouncing off to solve the EU issues on global fiscal deterioration.)

Anyway, the dietician agreed with what I was saying but had her protocols to follow, so, like Baldrick, I hatched a cunning plan. This involved my using the tube but telling the nurses that I was allowed a sloppy diet by the surgical team -which they accepted. So I was then in a position to say that the antibiotics were working, the tube was working, and I was able to eat without issue. Eventually, on Good Friday, I was seen by a surgical doctor who listened to my reasoning and what I had done over the previous day or so and agreed with me that I could be allowed to go home. I must point out here that again there were positive people on that ward: not everyone viewed me with the disdain Ms Ratchet hoped for. One such was a nurse, who dealt with my clinical appointments at Maidstone and was just temporarily on the ward, and the other was a nurse on my discharge day whose first day it was on that ward: they were lovely. Lastly, I should point out that there were five other patients on that ward, and, to be honest, their treatment was about on a par with mine, so I am unsure what they must have done: perhaps made some of the staff carry out those silly medical things that got in the way of their day.

Anyway, I was safely ensconced back on my sofa later that day and happy in the knowledge that I was out of there and that there were some seriously cheesy sci-fi films on over Easter. I should love to say that my issues over the feeding-tube were now finished, but alas, I cannot. Again it was the stitches, and the last one was when two of the three came out, and it was agreed that a doctor would come round to the chemo-ward during my third cycle and give me a quick stitch up. No, he didn't send me back to that ward whilst I had my chemo. Unfortunately, when I turned up for my chemo, I was advised that they didn't want to do this, as they wanted me to go back to Maidstone. Unfortunately both Sue, my specialist nurse, and Ashley, my dietician, who had put this in place, were off that Friday, so, after a call to the HEN team, I awaited their reply.

The outcome was that one surgeon had refused, but one had said he would do it, but only if I went round to A&E after my chemo, as all the tools for it were in place there. Well, I went to A&E only to discover that the said surgeon was not at Margate that day! One of his colleagues, however, stated that she was very busy but if I booked myself in she would get to me when she could. Well, based on my previous trips being from six hours to a few days, and after just having chemo-drugs pumped into me for the last eight hours, I politely declined. Unfortunately when the last stitch came out that evening, I knew that it would mean a trip to Maidstone or London, as it might now have dislodged from my duodenum, so I sent an email to Sue and Ashley, knowing they wouldn't see it till the Monday, and decided to cover the tube up as best I could and hope I had no eating issues over the next few days. Fortunately I didn't, so was rather happy that I had managed a full week without being admitted to a hospital.

The previous week I was admitted with what I can only describe as a bloody scare. I have always been wary of getting admitted to hospital, because sometimes I believe that I can control the problems better at home, but - and this is important - I will always do what the professionals say, and so should you. I may put my own alternative view across, I may procrastinate, but ultimately, if they tell you it needs sorting in the proper environment, you have to do as they say. They are qualified, we are not. The knowledge you have of your own circumstances is invaluable, but theirs has more foundation and depth. The reason for my latest excursion was that one of the main ongoing issues is the fact that I no longer have a stomach, just a pouch. This means that just one mouthful of food more than my body can take will result in a long slow pain that can be eased only with time and rest, or what I have eaten will come straight back up. Well, on this day, it did both, so I retired to bed, propped myself up and tried to distract myself with *Dinocroc vs Megasaurus*, a truly classic film. About an hour later, I felt sick again and returned to the great white orb, only to vomit a rather large blood-clot. After a few minutes of trying to work out whether it was just some discoloured food or whether I had retched too much and that had caused it, I realised it was indeed a blood-clot, and panic duly set in. I decided my best option was to contact my chemotherapy out-of-hours line, as they had all my details available and could best advise, although I really knew the outcome: A&E.

I convinced the nurse that, if I tried 111, they might send an on-call doctor, which she agreed I could try, but unfortunately they wanted the same. So they dispatched an ambulance, assuring me the ambulance would be with me in about half an hour and it would not be a blue-light job; they would assess me and then decide whether I needed to go into hospital. Ten minutes later, the street was lit up more brightly than Sydney Harbour Bridge on New Year, and all the neighbours were at their doors. Fortunately it missed my house and went down the street, only to reverse a few minutes later, minus the blue lights. After some tests, the inevitable happened, and I was on my way to Canterbury Hospital, a new venue for me.

After some tests and a move from A&E to CDU, I was put on a ward, where it was discovered I was slightly anaemic, and they wanted to do an endoscopy to see what was happening. This scared me more than the clot, because the last time I was anaemic and had an endoscopy was back in the Monty Python sketch at the very start of this book. When it turned out that it was a small bleed that had happened on one of my internal stitches from the main operation and appeared to have resolved itself, I was all good to go, with monitoring and a change to one of my medications. That was after they had done the two stitches that had come out during my stay. Well, the doctor did the replacement stitches, and I should have known when he mentioned that they only had certain sutures that were a little too thin that, as in the case of the guy in the massage-parlour with an empty wallet, this was not going to end well. The result was my needing the two stitches to be done again during my chemo, as previously mentioned.

Before I was discharged from Canterbury hospital, a surgical doctor took the time to come and redo my two missing stitches. I guess it didn't bode too well when he advised me that he didn't have access to the correct-sized stitches but would try and 'double up' and do his best. Unfortunately I went home, and the next day the stitches came out again. After speaking to Ashley, my dietician, A&E was mentioned again, but I pointed out that I was having chemotherapy the following Friday and that I had seen people have minor issues dealt with whilst there. So I asked whether it would be possible to have the stitches redone whilst I was having my chemotherapy treatment. Ashley agreed that this was the best option and said she would liaise with Sue, my specialist nurse, and arrange. Well, the appointed treatment-day came, and, as my arm was warmed up so the nurses could attempt to find a vein (bless them, by this time finding a vein in my arms was like finding hens' teeth), I was asked by one of the nurses whether 'I had managed to sort the stitches problem'. This was news to me, as I believed it to be all in place. However, it turned out that the same old issue of not wanting to touch the tube in certain hospitals had again raised its head. The surgical team had refused, and nothing was in plan. I tried to speak to Ashley and Sue, but they were off on that day, so I contacted the HEN team and asked them to chase the situation.

The outcome was that one surgeon at QEQM, where I was having my chemo treatment, had refused to touch the tube, but one surgeon had said he would re-stitch, but only if I went round to A&E after my chemo, as all the equipment he needed was there. Well, the nurses on the chemo-ward were fantastic and got my treatment finished a little early. I therefore headed round to A&E with an optimistic glint in my eye, just like Pinocchio hoping to become a 'real boy'. Oh, how misguided we both were! Apparently a recent survey said Pinocchio can lie only twelve times before he falls over! When I got to A&E, I was advised that the surgeon who said he would do my procedure was not working there that day, and, after some persuading of the reception-staff, they rang through. A surgeon told them that they were very busy but were aware of me. If I booked into the A&E department, I should be seen as soon as possible, but no guarantee. At this, I pointed out that I had just been having chemotherapy treatment for the last eight hours, and, although the prospect of spending several more in their department filled me with the joys of spring, I should politely decline their kind offer.

Once home, I decided a nice relaxing bath would soothe my day, but, instead, I soon noticed that the final stitch in my tube had given up the ghost, and the tube itself had come out a couple of inches. With the experience I now had of this piece of kit, I knew that it was redundant. The fact it had moved from its internal position by the duodenum meant no external stitches would be done. I mulled this over whilst trying to stifle a sniffle, like a five-year-old boy who knows he can't have the new bike but really thinks those big sobs will help, and decided that I would drop an email to Ashley and Sue. I knew they would not see it until Monday, which gave me the weekend to patch up and protect the tube-site and ensure I was able to eat as best I could so as to avoid any more hospital stays. The chemo kicked in, and my intake of food was reduced, but I felt I was getting enough into me not to warrant needing the feeding-tube. I therefore awaited the decision by the teams on the Monday.

The first email I received was from a dietician who would be taking over from Ashley in the next week or so, as Ashley was leaving her job after her one-year contract: again an issue over funding and permanency within positions. The email advised me of the fact that they had worked very hard to have my stitches done the previous Friday and that surgeons needed to prioritise workloads etc. I was quite surprised by this, as I was very aware that they had tried to resolve the situation, and I pointed out that I was aware that things needed to be prioritised. However, I went on, I just did not feel well enough to be in an A&E department for many hours. The irony is there to see.

The rest of the day was a succession of emails between various persons advising each other that they wanted the tube left in place or that I must go to an A&E, but at least they did copy me in on their deliberations, which was nice. Eventually on the Tuesday I was called by Sue; it was usually this kind lady who took the bull by the horns and tried to resolve things. After a long discussion, we agreed that the present tube was in fact redundant; that it would not be treated by any East Kent hospital; and that if it were to remain it would probably need to be replaced. I advised that, although my eating was reduced, I did not feel any serious concerns, so we agreed that the tube would be removed. Sue spoke to Michelle, my specialist surgical nurse at Maidstone, who, I must add, has been fantastic herself throughout all my problems, and I was booked into Maidstone to have the tube removed the next day. As it was already loose and there were no internal fixtures, this was simply a case of taking it out under controlled circumstances.

I arrived at Maidstone hospital the following day, which just happened to be the day that the report into the alleged surgical problems I mentioned previously had come out, and the chief executive was vigorously protesting against some of the points raised in it. So I was quite stunned, but realistically unsurprised, by what happened next. Michelle took me in to meet a surgeon (apologies, but I did not catch his name, or I should quote it), and the first question from his lips was, 'So why do you want the tube?' I looked round, but try as I might I just couldn't see a DeLorean that might have whisked me back to a previous appointment. He then examined the site and asked Michelle to go and get some dressings. I am going to be very honest and truthful now and advise you one very important thing. No matter how much you feel indebted to a member of the medical profession, no matter how much you think they know best, if you are alone with someone having treatment and you feel uncomfortable, stop the appointment and ask to wait until someone else is present. Most people will assume that I am going to go into some form of Operation-Yewtree mode, but I am not. This is what happened and trust me: I feel it is just as important.

Once Michelle had left the room, he started attempting to feed the tube back into me; by this time it had come out six or seven inches. As you can imagine, this was quite painful, so I asked him to please stop. He ignored me and continued to play with the tube as if it were something on the latest top ten Christmas toy list and he couldn't quite work out why. He again tried to push the tube back into me, and I again asked him to stop, pointing out that I believed the appointment was to remove the tube. He must have then got bored: he decided to pull it out, with no warning, all the while looking at it in wonder and declaring that he 'had no idea it was so long'! He took the tube that he had just removed from my body and threw it in a normal bin as if it was the wrapper from his lunch. In case you are unaware, I believe that all medical waste should go into a yellow bin.

At this point Michelle returned and dressed the site. She was again very supportive and told me to make contact if I had any further problems. It was probably a few hours later that what had happened started to sink in and make me quite angry, but after the dismissive and indirect emails from previously that week I decided that it would probably be seen as just another moan and that I need not mention it. I consoled myself with the knowledge that I should not have to deal with Maidstone Hospital again but inwardly cringed. Whilst the hospital's boss was defending it quite verbally outside, it was business as usual for his staff inside.

I must say here, though, that the nurses and staff on the ward, in particular at Canterbury, were fantastic. There were issues and problems, but they were down to the same old story of one nurse having far too much to do. Herein lies the issue. I said I should not get political about the NHS, and I shan't, because different parties have tried different ways to 'improve' the service over the years, and all have failed as far as I can see. What I have seen over my dealings with the NHS is that the emphasis has been moved from care to finance. The basics no longer seem to matter, and as a result the service seems to be on the edge of a rather large cliff. A&E departments are being strangled by targets to deal with patients that, if they are missed, can see them being fined up to the salary of one nurse in some cases: their departments being swamped by people who are more likely to use the service, justifiably or not, and a plethora of patients that simply cannot get appointments at their doctors' surgeries. On hospital wards the rule is, I believe, one nurse to eight patients maximum. This is regularly the case and is fine if a nurse is dealing with eight patients with minor conditions. However, when they are dealing with eight patients who have serious conditions, just one patient having a bad day can mean the other seven see no form of proper care, and I must stress that this is not the nurses' fault. I must add also that at no time did I feel unsafe.

Another thing I have seen and discussed with people in the profession is the fact that this often results in the staff on wards and in other departments not staying. You then have a situation where the NHS is paying double, sometimes triple, the shift wage to someone who many times appears to be, and often is, just there for the money. Permanent positions are often advertised at salaries below a reasonable amount for their responsibility, meaning they are not taken up, so the NHS then employ more locums to fill the positions, again at double the cost. There is also the good old mantra of slowly secretly and discreetly privatising many parts. They say it is for efficiency, but it usually means that some rich old school-tie-run company picks up a very lucrative contract that in no way benefits the NHS, and the relevant departments are forced to work to tighter budgets, which makes more cash for the new owners, totally undermining the principles on which the NHS was formed.

I have gone on in this chapter about some of the issues I faced in my experience, as they are an important part of what I went through and they need to be included for me to write a book that gives a full picture of my dealing with this awful disease. I know it is risky, and some may view me as negative, but it is all true and honest. It is cathartic for me to write it, and I hope that it gives you a sense of where things can go wrong in the hope you can resolve any issues better and more quickly to aid your own treatment. I am also aware, after discussions with many nurses, that I really did probably just have a run of bad luck for a lot of the problems. Who is to say that my bad day didn't tie in with someone else's to create a situation that might otherwise not have happened?

The main feeling I have toward the NHS is extreme gratitude. Yes, there have been issues that I really believe are not right. I have been asked whether I wished to complain, and the closest I came was with Ms Ratchet. Even then I did not believe she was a real danger to patients, so I did not wish to. I do not believe in taking away anything from a beloved system that has faults but is genuinely trying to work to its original principles of real care and best treatment. 99.99% of people in the NHS are there because it's their vocation. They care, and they work hard to qualify to be able to do that. They are often restricted, overworked, stressed and downright depressed with the system they have to endure day in day out, but they continue to try to give the best they can. They deal with and see things on a daily basis that would leave most people in a state, but they cope the best they can and come back the very next day to do it all again. My biggest worry for the NHS is how long these people will continue to put up with this relentless situation, or is that the government's plan? Attrition, apathy, then in for the kill. I certainly hope not, because the NHS is a wonderful institution that is unique to our country and should be there working under its founding principles for decades to come. One way we can try our best to help is to keep a close eye on our dealings with it; monitor news and changes and voice our opinions. If we all jump together, they will hear the thump.

Chapter Ten

The Operation – Oesophagectomy

My operation was booked for first thing Tuesday 7 January 2014. I was to arrive at St Thomas' Hospital London the day before at around 3pm; they say to settle you in and get all the paperwork done, but I think it's so you can't have any last-minute changes of mind and bolt for the nearest airport. I took the train up on the Monday, and the only thing I can remember is thinking I was going to treat myself to a McDonald's meal at Waterloo Station: a strange sort of last meal, but, as I knew what was coming, some crap food was just what I needed. The only problem was, instead of going for my normal Big Mac meal, I went for one of their new ones and didn't quite enjoy it. It was a strange feeling being in a London train-station, with my suitcase, knowing where I was going, whilst others with similar were hopefully going somewhere much nicer: unless it was somewhere with a serious food-hygiene problem where they might get jealous of my having my stomach removed. I then decided to take a nice slow walk the ten minutes or so it would take me to get from the station to the hospital. By this point the nerves were starting to set in, and a myriad negative thoughts were running through my mind. When I had had my appointment with Professor Mason a couple of weeks previously, I had expected a survival percentage as you see on TV and in the films:

'I can only give you a 20% chance of survival, Mr Quinn.'

'So better odds than my having sex before the op then. That's good!'

The reality is, in my case, that it never happened: the percentage, not the sex bit. What the good professor did tell me was that the operation was one of the most serious and intrusive they do in this country, and on a scale of 1 to 10 it was about a 9. So as you can imagine I was pretty nervous walking up to the hospital. It was almost like being on one of those conveyor belts you see on cartoons where you are helpless as you head towards twenty different types of blades but your brain keeps trying to calm you by saying that the hero will press the big red stop-button at the last second. Again, though, in my case, a sense of inevitability overtook me, and I began to accept that it was quite simple: I should survive or I shouldn't.

The first thing that hit me as I walked into St Thomas' was just how vast it is: shops, restaurants, banks, a cinema and hundreds of people shuffling through it all. For a second I thought I might have got lost and ended up at Bluewater shopping-centre, but then I realised Bluewater doesn't have signs directing you to the operating theatres. I went up to my assigned ward and was directed to my bed and told by the nice nurse that I could have some time to myself and to take a walk round the hospital if I wanted, as long as I was back by 6 when some of the doctors might want to see me. This struck me as a bit strange, as I had envisaged being admitted, then being immediately hooked up to all sorts of wires and tubes and even a machine that went 'bing'.

Only fourteen people work in my office, and I was here to have a major operation. At about the same odds as winning the lottery, one of my colleagues was at the same hospital at the same time having a serious operation as well! Martin was having an op on his heart-valves, and so I took a wander round to the part of the hospital that he was in to say hello. I had a chat with him and was pleased to hear he would be allowed home the next day, which was great for him as he had spent a lot of time in hospital waiting for his operation, but it also was encouraging for me, as he had had his op only five days previously. The reason I say this is again the confusion created by Maidstone Hospital. Originally, as I have said, they were talking about my being in hospital for quite some considerable time; they even talked of up to two weeks in intensive care post-op as a precaution, which conflicted with the information I had been given by St Thomas'. However after reading the report on the problems at Maidstone, I understood the confusion, as I believe that one of the issues addressed was a kind of procrastination at Maidstone in moving patients forward in their recovery. St Thomas' were completely the opposite, as I was about to find out. I wished Martin all the best, left him to take a wander round the hospital and then headed back up to my ward.

One of the things that I have mentioned and I found a worry was the lack of consistency with things, mainly due to the involvement of different hospitals and trusts. This may be particular to my case, but one of them came about that evening. As I sat on the ward in my pjs doing a crossword, whist convincing myself the answer to 7 down couldn't really be 'incision,' I was approached by a man considerably younger than I am who introduced himself as Mr Gossage, my surgeon. My immediate reaction was rising panic: nothing to do with this gentleman but because, after the Maidstone débâcle of 2013, my nerves and worries had been settled by my meeting Professor Mason. Where was my consistency of treatment? Where was the patient-surgeon relationship that all films and TV had promised me? Where was the door? The trouble is that you think all these things but get swept up by the conversation you are having, and your old friend Acceptance starts to massage your brain. So I sat talking to the good doctor whilst trying to control my panic as it raged in my chest. However, whether it was Mr Gossage's great nature or the fact that the panic in my chest had to fight for space with an 11cm tumour I am unsure, but I started to calm down and to listen to what he was telling me. Up until this point, I knew that the tumour would be removed along with the infected lymph-nodes beside it in my stomach, but what I had no clue about was quite how much of my stomach would be removed. As Mr Gossage explained with words and diagrams, like some extreme version of the plan being put forward on Junk Yard Wars, it really began to sink in why this operation was described as major and intrusive. The plan was to remove the cancerous parts; then, like some strange scene cut from Apollo 13, to use what was left of my stomach to make a new oesophagus. This would leave me with a pouch instead of a stomach but, more importantly, with the cancer removed. As I sat through that evening seeing a procession of doctors and nurses and signing various consent forms, the importance of my situation really hit home, and, as I looked at the other patients in the ward and the worried faces on their loved ones, I felt very scared and very alone. Perhaps, this was my farewell.

I awoke the next morning, quite early, thinking it was the worry or nerves, only to be disappointed: it was the lady nurse or doctor typing away at an ancient NHS computer that I think had the keyboard from an old telex machine. The strange thing is, though, despite everything, I felt very positive for some reason. Again I think my brain had taken over, and after all I had been lucky to be there, and this was just the next stage in my holiday with Mr C. The only thing that was worrying me was whether I should be able to do no.2 before they took me down. Now this may seem strange to some, but throughout all my routines (and probably after the great iodine table incident of '09) I always made sure I had gone to the toilet before anaesthetic, as I was convinced if I didn't Mr Hankey would end up standing on the operating table beside me shouting 'Hi de ho'.

That morning saw another procession of doctors and descriptions, to the point I was looking forward to getting knocked out, but preferably not by the nurse whose fantastic chest I couldn't help staring at. My time came, and I was wheeled down to the operating theatre, and again I was struck by how vast this place was. I must have passed a dozen theatres before they wheeled me into the little room adjoining mine where the anaesthetist and his team were waiting for me. I knew I was going to be getting an epidural, and I was aware it can sometimes be painful, so I started looking round for the even smaller room where I was given anaesthetic to relieve the pain for getting my anaesthetic. Unfortunately for me the doctor got the needle so far in, but it would not take, so he had to do it again whilst I sat with my chin as far on to my chest as I could, trying to be all stoic, as there really were some pretty ladies in the room. Eventually it took, and I heard the longed-for words, 'You'll soon find yourself drifting off now, Mr Quinn.' This was just before 9am, and the next thing I remember was realising just how Darth Vadar must have felt when he came round. It was about 9pm when they brought me round, and, after the initial confusion, I was suddenly aware of all the tubes and lines coming out of me. That didn't really faze me until I started to wonder exactly where they were all going!

It was quite strange lying in the recovery-room feeling odd but not in pain (yet!). All I could do was watch the various nurses walk around and try not to get too fixated on the worried faces of the partners of other patients in the room. the previous evening I had met a chap called George who was having the same type of surgery as me, and his partner very kindly came over to see how I was doing, but, being more dosed up than Charlie Sheen on a Friday night, I think I just burbled something incoherent and went back to visual drifting. It was about this time I got to experience first-hand what some of our nurses and doctors have to put up with, as for about an hour the mood in the recovery-room was dictated (absolutely the right word to use) by a complete dick. All anyone could hear was this bloke screaming and shouting, threatening and swearing at anyone who came near him. I asked the nurse whether it was a road accident or such, (praying she wouldn't say it was some idiot who had just been given a replacement feeding tube but for some unknown reason he was pretending it hurt !!! As my Maidstone experiences had not quite left my short term memory) only to be told he was a regular drug-user on his third overdose that week; pleasant chap.

Eventually George and I were wheeled up to the high-dependency ward, which was a four-bedded room with a couple of dedicated nurses and various other people coming and going, but for me the best thing bar none was the view from my window of the Palace of Westminster, although I don't think the nurse and I got off on the right foot when asked whether She wanted to see Big Ben? Whilst tugging on my bed sheet. The only thing I really remember about that first night was meeting a pain-nurse. Yes, that really is a specific role, but unfortunately she doesn't wear black leather and ask questions whilst cracking the whip. This was to see where you were on the 'pain scale' and to set you up with your own little morphine-releasing button. The pain scale, which I had come across before, is where they ask you to rate your pain from 1 to 10, 1 being the least and 10 being the worst you had ever experienced. I had a think and selected a firm 7: I was still covered by the earlier anaesthetic and epidural, but I did feel the pain-level starting to creep upwards. The thing to bear in mind about this scale is, again, it is the individual's own tolerance, and some can handle more than others, just as with drink and other things. I have to say, however, the highest I ever scored was after they put my second feeding-tube in much later in that recovery-room at Maidstone, when I scored a 9. The reason I mention this is really aimed at the blokes, and I may cause controversy here, but for years I had put 'man 'flu' as a serious 7, but in reality it didn't even warrant a 1. However, after all this, I think it will creep back up to at least a 6. I tried epidural, ladies: you try man 'flu!

A point I need to let all you independent people out there know arose when I had been in the high-dependency ward for a few hours. A simple thing, or so I thought, was that, with more tubes in me than Dr Frankenstein's latest experiment, I was, needless to say, quite uncomfortable at times. My natural instinct was to attempt to shuffle myself up and down the bed to try and get more settled. It was as I tried this that the nurse-in-charge came over with a face only just sterner than the big lady on *The Chase* and scowled at me, stating that, if I needed to move or rearrange my bed, I should let her know so that she could do it. I felt this was a little harsh and didn't think I warranted such a chastising, but she went on to say that, at such a vital time in recovery, it was important that the nurses knew of any issues and that I could easily do more damage to myself at this stage than a

70s' DJ asking an undercover Yewtree operative to look at his old backstage pictures. The fact is that, unimportant as things may seem, you must put your faith and your trust in these professionals. I know it goes against the grain when you have spent your whole adult life fending for yourself, but there is always a point to their methods - unlike *The Voice*.

One of the things that surprised me (and I believe it was a point of failing in Maidstone) was how pro-active St Thomas' hospital was. In the afternoon after the op, I was approached by a couple of nurses who were part of the physiotherapy team and, before I realised what was happening, they had me swinging my legs over the side of the bed and then standing. I was surprised by the fact they were asking this of me so soon after the operation, but more so that I was able to, even if I did look like some weird cyborg with all my tubes! They also gave me some light exercise routines to do, which were pretty basic and involved raising my arms to shoulder-height and then standing and raising my knees about twenty times. These exercises were certainly not easy, but the nurses did not force me as if in some weird fetish scenario. However, the exercises are very important in recovery after such serious operations, as they reduce the risk of a lot of complications, such as fluid's being retained in the lungs. At this point I started to think I should be home by the weekend, such was my optimism in what I was able to do after such serious surgery. Whatever the reason, I certainly found this to be a positive thing.

With regard to the tubes coming and going about my person, I should explain what they were all for. I obviously had a cannula, which allows the nurses to administer drugs etc. without the need for an injection each time. I had two chest drains, which allow any fluid around the chest to drain into a large tub which needed to be carried around, and also I had a catheter. This latter engendered a weird feeling, especially when you realise you are having a pee while the attractive nurse is discussing the serious side of post-operative complications with you. I felt a lot like Steve Martin's character in Dirty Rotten Scoundrels. The last tube I had was the feeding-tube that would cause me many problems in the months to come. So you see, I wasn't exaggerating. The reason for the feeding-tube is that, after operations where physical changes have been made to the digestive system, the site needs five days to be able to repair itself before any food or liquid can be ingested. After five days they send you for an x-ray. You have to swallow a horrid drink that contains absolutely no alcohol, and, if there are no leaks, you can progress to the next stage of eating. The stages I went through were: nothing for five days; then I was allowed some ice to suck for a couple of days; then what they call a 'wet diet,' which was soups and ice cream etc; after that came a soft diet: this was things like mince and scrambled eggs; until finally you are able to eat most things - a bit like the Kate Moss diet of 2004. This is dependent on the individual's recovery, but I managed to request my first soft meal of scrambled eggs on toast after seven days. I should have taken heed when the lady taking my order asked me whether I was sure, so I shouldn't have been surprised when the eggs finally arrived the next morning with more powder in them than Nelson's flagship.

On the subject of hospital food - and bear in mind I have had the great pleasure of eating out at most of these fine establishments - I have to say that I found it all very good on the whole. There was, of course, the odd exception, but the food was usually pretty appetising. I cannot, however, give a 100% endorsement, as most of the stays I had in hospital were usually down to eating issues or infections, so it was usually on the day before discharge that I got to choose a meal I wanted. I have to add, though, that the nicest thing to pass my lips was on day six after my main operation, when I was given a polystyrene cup filled with crushed ice cubes: absolute bliss!

After a day on the high-dependency ward, I was moved round to my permanent ward, and the first thing I felt was quite depressed, as I had gone from having a lovely view from my window to being in the middle bay of three beds with nothing to see but blue curtains. It's quite surprising how such a small thing can bring you down, but, when you are all hooked up and have little or no mobility, just having a view can be a life-saver. I was very lucky, though, as one of the doctors noticed this, and after a chat she had me moved to another bay next to the window. Now obviously not every patient can be lucky enough to have a window-bay, but I think they realised I should be in there a lot longer than others. I believe that's why I was moved.

I then got on with the slow process of healing. I was pretty good at keeping up my exercise-routine and after a few days was up to taking a walk round the ward. The only real issue I had in those first few days was getting the balance of pain medication right. My epidural was removed after day two on the permanent ward, as it had started to come out anyway, but I was on a combination of slow-release morphine twice a day and the highest allowed rate on my self-administering pump. The result of this was that I was keeping the pain at bay but almost always on the verge of sleep. Slowly we lowered the amounts to a point where I was keeping the pain under control but still not quite like the front bench of the House of Commons during a debate on the pork percentage of sausages.

As time went by, I got to various stages where some of the invading army of tubes could be removed, like some human détente. The first to come out was my catheter, and I was more worried than a hedge-fund manager at Lehman Brothers. However, although it was a sensation I should not care to repeat, it wasn't painful, and just to be peeing, even if into a recycled container, was a small slice of heaven on a plate. The next to come out was one of my chest-drains, and this one did worry me, for the following reasons. Now I shall try not to be judgemental here, but a patient came in a few days after my arrival having had an appendectomy. He soon made himself a popular member of the ward with gems such as, 'I know I should have gone private, papa, but I didn't have much choice, being unconscious. Anyway, it's pretty rough, and the nurses don't fill me with confidence, but I should be home tomorrow.' Or who could forget the old classic to a nurse checking his dressings: 'So you're from Australia, are you? Don't they have enough proper nurses here anymore?' Or my personal favourite: 'I really shall be having a word with my local MP, as the standard of nursing in here is really quite appalling.' I couldn't decide whether he was an ignorant buffoon or really so arrogant, talentless and spoilt that he had lost all contact with reality: a sort of male Katie Price.

However, the reason the chap in the bay next to me and I were slightly worried about having our drain-tubes removed was that Rupert the Nob, as I shall refer to him for now, had his taken out the previous day, and I can only say that the last time I saw drama like that it was Shakespearean, and the last time I heard a scream of such a high pitch it was coming from someone whose testes were still hanging on to their stomach and refusing to budge, like the world's worst parachutist. Even though having a cannula put in can be quite a sore experience, if you have veins like mine, which are more regressed than the Amish, it is just that: sore; not excruciating. So when Rupert the Nob yelped like a mistreated dog when his was put in, I should have borne that in mind regarding the removal of his drain-tube. It was, however, with some trepidation I was chosen to precede the chap in the bay next to me for having it removed. As I lay on my side with one nurse grasping the tube firmly (gosh, I get some weird thoughts at some inappropriate times) and another nurse offering to hold my hand, I prepared for the worst. Fortunately the removal was about as climactic as this paragraph: a very weird sensation, but no pain, just a millisecond of discomfort. The chap in the bay next to me was quite stunned and now optimistic about his own removal, but best of all was Rupert asking the nurse why his tube must have been longer to cause him so much pain and why he couldn't have had a smaller one like me. Innuendos ran round my head as the nurse, also with a quite satisfied grin on her face, answered Rupert: 'Mr Quinn's was about a foot and a half longer than yours and was in much deeper!' Sadly Rupert left us shortly after that. Only to go back to planet 'Made in Chelsea'. Sadly.

The days went by, and I slowly began to recover. I upped my walking regime and slowly started to feel a lot less pain. I was taken off the self-administering morphine button after a week, which was like seeing your grandma go home after a visit: you know she has to go, but, boy, will you miss the treats! I had a few visitors over my stay, despite my saying that there was no need. I wasn't trying to be the heroic type - fat chance - but it was purely because I was in London, and it was quite a journey to make for the ones who did visit. I was a little miffed, though, when I read the various Facebook pages stating how they were 'off to visit Mr Quinn' and then taking full advantage of being in London, leaving me and heading to a nice pub on the riverside!

One of the things that irked me during my stay was the cost of watching the TV. Not all hospitals have the facility for patients to watch telly by their bedside, but St Thomas' did. You have this little movable screen and some headphones, and you can disappear into *Homes under the Hammer* whilst Rupert the Nob screams as they remove a plaster. The trouble is it is quite expensive, about £20 for three days. I had read somewhere that even prisoners get telly cheaper than this, so it was with a grudge as big as David Milliband's handing over a Christmas card to his brother that I ended up spending about £60 during my stay. One of my friends Kev, works for the prison service, and by coincidence he was doing guard-duty over a long-term patient in the same ward as me and came to visit me a couple of times. I took consolation that at least this prisoner would be paying the same rate as me, but alas, I was informed that his family had bought him a TV. I consoled myself with the fact that my lovely sister had bought me a Kindle Fire, and at least I should be taking mine home in the foreseeable future.

As time went by and my healing continued, I eventually had the remaining drain and staples removed - all sixty-eight of them, and at this point we were looking at my being discharged. I have always been quite proactive about my leaving hospital, but I was acutely aware that this was slightly different, as the importance of the operation and the fact I live alone loomed large in my mind. So with that in mind I showed the nurses and doctors I was keen to get home but also cautious and accepting of their advice, as the worst thing that I could have done was find myself at home regretting being there if it was too soon.

The one thing that saved me from having to make a decision too soon was that I needed a procedure to have the temporary feeding-tube changed from a catheter to the proper jejunostomy tube, and I was due for it on a Friday, which meant I should probably be discharged on the Saturday. Unfortunately, or fortunately, depending on your viewpoint, on the day in question the department due to perform this procedure was extremely busy, the result being they could not fit me in until the following Tuesday. So like a groom whose bride doesn't turn up, I had a stay of execution.

One thing I must mention about my stay at St Thomas' was the nursing staff. Again there were some issues, usually around stressed nurses doing too many shifts and hours, so not being the most sympathetic. There were also the temp-agency night-nurses who had as much interest in the patients as the Lorry driver delivering the clean laundry!. However for the last week or so I was there, I had the loveliest two nurses looking after me. One was Australian, and one was from New Zealand, but I won't hold their convict status against them. (I wonder whether their families bought them a TV.) These two girls (they were both young) were absolutely what you would hope for in a nurse: genuinely caring and sympathetic, but with a strict side (easy, boys) and with a wit and knowledge that gave me complete trust in them. Susie and Lauren, I thank you both dearly.

One thing I must advise is that during this time things may be said or told to you by doctors and nurses that may, for some reason, not seem that important at the time but are. You may not get their gravity for various reasons, such as too much pain medication, or you may just not be having the greatest day, or, in my case, it may be being told to you by Nurse Hannibal who makes it more about her than you, so you do not get the importance. With me, the self-appointed champion of all that is medical knowledge was charged with the task of giving me the results of my surgery. I had seen Mr Gossage at various stages of my stay, and he was extremely happy with the way the operation had gone and advised me that they believed they had managed to extract all the tumour and its associated elements, and they were distinctly positive for my future. However, it was down to Hannibal to advise me of the technical results of the operation. The fact that the first five minutes of our chat consisted of her handing me a booklet on possible side-effects and how to cope with the physical changes to my body from the op, and then advising me how she had been instrumental in writing said booklet took my mind away from what she was saying. She then tried to get me to join a coffee-group of people who had gone through my type of surgery,

which met twice a week, and told me it would help me. I pointed out to her that I lived in Dover, not round the corner from the meetings in London, and again this point seemed lost on her as she looked at me as if I had just been handed the keys to the universe and passed them straight back.

The upshot was that when she took the thirty seconds she set aside to inform me of my results, I was not very receptive. Fortunately I realised the importance of this information later and asked my surgeon to go through it again with me, and the result was that there were some areas around the new internal joins that they were monitoring, but the chemo had worked better than expected and, of thirty-one lymph-nodes tested, only two had any cancerous activity (and apparently anything less than three is great news). It now seemed that I might be leaving St Thomas' without half my stomach but also without my cancer. I had the feeding-tube changed on the Tuesday and was discharged the following day. It was a long day, but I eventually got home, thanks to a kindly sister who arranged patient-transport for me, at about 8pm. Exhausted, nervous and slightly afraid, I settled myself in for my recovery period. I had some friends visit over the next few days; I got all my prescriptions delivered; and thank goodness there is online food-shopping nowadays. So all I needed to do was relax, rest and get myself ready for the next batch of chemo and my eventual return to normality. As you have already read, I was about as close to the mark on that one as Tony Blair was on WMD.

Chapter Eleven

It's My Party, and I'll Cry If I Want To

When I first thought about writing this book, I had a vague plan in my head of how it would read and what I wanted to get across. I didn't start writing it until I had been to St Thomas' and had my oesophagetomy, so I was pretty confident that I would be able to finish it, unlike the times I visited female friends after a day at the pub! It is therefore quite a shock to find myself now writing this chapter, as it is not one that I had even considered would need to be written. I mentioned previously that Sue, the specialist nurse at QEQM, had forewarned me about the possibility I might struggle when I received my all-clear, but I had no idea how much and how true this warning would be. I don't believe I am weaker or stronger than any other person who might find themselves dealing with cancer, but this is what happened to me, and I write it to forewarn any that may experience the same.

'After reviewing your CT scan, we can find no cancerous cells in your body.'

This was the sentence that was delivered to me by Dr Waters, my oncologist, at Canterbury Hospital on Wednesday 28 May 2014. The smile on Dr Waters' face and the nurse standing beside him emphasised the words a little more. Unlike my diagnosis, this information was accepted by my brain immediately. I cannot say whether that was because it was fantastic news or whether it was because of the course of treatment I had, that I was almost expecting it, after all, and, as previously mentioned, they would not operate if they didn't think they could get it all. I let the words wash over me like the applause and feel of the outstretched tape at the finishing line of some major race. (I have to use my imagination here, as I have not experienced that feeling, to be honest, but I don't think a polite ripple after coming second at the Inter-School discus competition of '81 quite gives the moment the same impetus!)

We then discussed how things would progress from there. I was now classed as cancer-free and was in the five-year watch-and-monitor stage. I expected to hear the word 'remission' but didn't. I guess that word is only said to people who have had the type of cancer that wasn't a physical lump like my tumour: the type that is beaten by drugs alone or by radiotherapy, and I suppose the worry is of its reappearing - which would be as welcome as Gary Glitter on a 70s revival tour. I was to see Dr Waters every three months for the upcoming future, and I believe that it then would drop to six months, then annually. I left Canterbury Hospital in a slight daze that day, which is understandable, I suppose. I told my sister and a few close friends and let the wider community know via Facebook. Things were definitely looking up. I received a bottle of champagne from the MD at work and I was due to visit my sister and brother-in-law the following weekend. It just so happened that my sister and some of her work-colleagues were doing the Race for Life 5k run in support of Cancer Research when I was visiting, so being able to pop the cork on the champagne after they had all crossed the line seemed very poignant and fitting; just slightly annoyed they expected me then to share it with them!

The day of that race was very emotional for me, as you can imagine. Being in such close proximity not just to people who had survived cancer but also to the families and friends of those people, and unfortunately also of people who had not survived. They had a large board where people could post short comments, and to read the devastating outcomes some families had gone through mentioned again and again is very humbling.

After my visit, I returned home feeling exhausted but optimistic and happy. Physically I was still very weak from the operation, and there were issues I was trying to deal with that I have not mentioned so far. I wondered whether to put these in a chapter headed 'Post-Op' but concluded that they would fit better in here - said Jessica, née Bill, to his new boyfriend. The main problems I was having were eating-issues and pain in the rib-area. The eating-issues were expected and separate from the issues I was having with the feeding-tube. Simply dealing with the fact that you no longer have a stomach is a major problem (said Ms Curry). One of the major difficulties was that I now had to embrace the 'little and often' eating regime: quite simply my stomach was gone, and in its place was a 'pouch' that the surgeon had made to replace it. No, I hadn't decided to become a surrogate mother to a Joey: as I have said, the surgery meant that I had been rearranged like someone with two toilet-roll innards, some double-sided tape and a coat-hanger in the strangest episode of Blue Peter ever transmitted. The first issue I encountered was reflux: no, not the Duran Duran song, but quite simply I no longer had a valve between my stomach (pouch) and mouth, so, if I was silly enough to overeat, any excess would simply come back up. I must point out that this is not the same as vomiting, but it is very worrying at first and also very unpleasant. The valve I refer to is the one where you would normally get heartburn or indigestion, if you suffer from such things. I believe this is the case, but they didn't quite go into such details on my First Aid at Work courses. You get informed of things like this, and other possible issues you may encounter, in the literature you receive on discharge from hospital, but literature is literature until you start to experience these problems. Personally I was just happy I had not suffered one such issue called 'Early/Late Dumping Syndrome.' Yes, that really is a possible side-effect, and I'm sure it is self-explanatory, but, in case you wonder, it doesn't mean trying to beat the queues at your local council tip.

I also went through problems with vomiting as well (hence I differentiate between the two). There were many periods that I can only compare myself with someone suffering from bulimia. I would eat, then it would come back up; I would eat again, and it would come back up – and so on. This wasn't me forcing myself to vomit in the unhinged psychological belief it would improve my body image (bearing in mind my torso was now beginning to resemble a map of train lines that Dr Beeching had deemed surplus to requirements): this was just something that was happening. It was almost like throwing a tin of paint at a wall in the hope that a brush-full would stick. This went on for a few weeks, and, after a few consultations with various medical staff, it was decided that I would need a procedure called a pyloric dilatation. This procedure involved an endoscopy with an extra attachment: 'free, and yours for just £5.99 plus £134.50 delivery here on the Home Medical Shopping Channel.' It would go through my newly-arranged pipe-work and gently widen things so that food could pass through more comfortably and not fester in my pouch and pipes like some unattended chemistry experiment. The first time I had this procedure done was at Maidstone Hospital, and at the same time they refitted my feeding-tube, but, owing to the aforementioned issues with that, I didn't get to realise any benefits of the procedure initially. I have since had it done again, but at St Thomas' and by Mr Gossage, the surgeon who performed my main operation, and I learned a couple of things from him before that one. I did get to feel the benefits almost immediately afterwards, either because Maidstone had done a half-hearted job previously or because of the issues they caused post-procedure. Either way, this seemed like the first time it had been done.

Also a major worry to me was the symptoms that pre-warn a dilatation is required. Apart from the vomiting, there is a pain in the chest and the eating problems mentioned, and every time I experienced them, I could not help but think back to the symptoms that led to my original diagnosis. I was quite terrified that the tumour was growing back and was going to hack its way out of me shouting, 'Here's Johnny!' It was only after talking to Mr Gossage prior to my second dilatation (the first one performed by him) that he explained why these symptoms were happening. Narrow passage, large volume means pain, again like the corridors backstage of a Jeremy Kyle show.

The other major issue I was having was that during my oesophagectomy the surgical team had broken one of my ribs on purpose (perhaps I shouldn't have made that joke about their fitting me in between golf-rounds), and it had subsequently not healed correctly. This now meant that I was experiencing quite a lot of pain from the rib-area, which was exacerbated by the rib's 'clicking' regularly every time I moved too much - a little like the clicking sensation you get in a knee when you stand sometimes. This really was a major problem for me, as it affected my mobility and my sleeping, to the point where, living at the top of six flights of stairs with no lift, I sometimes could not even leave the flat for fear of being unable to get back up said stairs.

The situation with the rib was really my biggest problem, but, from the first time I mentioned it to Mr Gossage on my visit a couple of weeks after the operation and for many months to come, I was told that this kind of fracture was indeed very painful and difficult to heal, but would eventually fix itself. This, as I say, went on for some months, and reasons such as the chemotherapy were put forward as explanations as to why it still had not healed; and I accepted them. It was only on a routine appointment with my GP months later, when I was told to be aware that it may never heal, that I thought, 'No, I can't put up with this for the rest of my life.' The residual pain I could learn to deal with. After all, I know, and I'm sure you know, friends who put up with pain of various types in their day-to-day life. What I didn't think I could put up with, however, was the constant clicking that multiplied the pain. I had tried gentle walking and even tried swimming to see whether it would help, but alas, to no avail. It was then that I started speaking to the oncology team and the surgical team to see whether anything could be done about it. It was after some badgering that I received an appointment with the surgical team at St Thomas' to discuss my options and went to meet a surgeon whom I had not met before, who was very sympathetic and understanding but felt that there wasn't much that could be done. He would, however, confer with the other surgeons in the department and see whether there was an option open to me. I tried to stress to him that it was the clicking that I just needed to stop.

Whilst I was waiting for the result of this meeting, I had the dilatation I previously mentioned with Mr Gossage at St Thomas', and, after discussing the procedure, he obviously noticed the discomfort and pain I was in with the rib and said he would look into it straight away and would get me operated on sooner rather than later. They could do an exploratory operation and see what the issue was and hopefully resolve it. The relief I felt was extreme, and quite frankly if there had been a department at St Thomas' that could have given me a uterus, I would quite happily have had that done and borne Mr Gossage's children.

So these were the physical problems I was experiencing when I received the news from Dr Waters about my all-clear. There were other problems, such as lethargy, fatigue and anxiety, but I kept being told that these were quite normal considering that my post-op recovery had been anything but routine and predictable. What I wasn't prepared for, despite my specialist nurse Sue's having warned me, was an all-encompassing sense of loss and bewilderment that hit me shortly after receiving this amazing news and returning from my sister's. I was aware how quickly the support-mechanisms can evaporate around you once an issue is considered resolved by the NHS, as I had learnt this when I finally did have my feeding-tube removed. All the nutritional support I had been receiving from the HEN team was gone in an instant. It makes perfect sense as I no longer had the tube, but there were still issues, and, although I was introduced to a dietician who called me every now and then to check up on me, I missed the general sense of support that having a telephone number or email address that you can use and know it will be a sympathetic and supportive reply gave me. What Sue tried to forewarn me about and what I really experienced was a huge sense of loss as the apparatus and infrastructure that had been around me for the last ten months was systematically withdrawn from me. I went from many appointments in a week, sometimes, to practically nothing. Yes, there were ongoing problems that were being looked at, but the main structure around me had been dismantled, a bit like having a session in the toilet because you need to go but when you come out someone has taken the whole house down around you.

Now I'm not moaning about this like some villain in a panto (oh, yes, you are!). It makes absolute sense that the infrastructure that was there to support and hopefully cure you of the cancer would disappear once it had met its objective. The NHS has limited funds and needs to spend them appropriately, unlike an MP on a freebie trip abroad to forge cultural links. Also the last thing I wanted to do was to take any form of asset away from people who were going through cancer in the NHS, be it financial or simply the time of medical staff. What I was not prepared for and what I did struggle with was an overwhelming feeling of isolation. It's difficult to explain, as Professor Hawkins said when a colleague thought his book, *A Brief History of Time*, was about male underwear through the ages; but the thing is that when you are embroiled in the rollercoaster of cancer, two things happen, or at least they did in my case. Firstly, and maybe this is just because of the form my treatment took, I was focused on issues as they arose. I was diagnosed, so, yes, that's happened; now let's focus on whether it has spread. It hasn't spread, great. Now let's focus on the procedures to find out its extent. Right, now we know its extent, let's see whether the chemotherapy will make it operable; and so on. I always focused on the next thing, a bit like Zsa Zsa Gabor for husband no.12. This form of focus kept me positive and also helped me to understand and accept things as they happened to me. I cannot say that you will feel the same regarding this, but as I keep repeating, it is very dependent on your type of cancer, your treatment-plan and of course you.

Whilst I was dealing with things this way and going through the treatment-plan, I was constantly being examined, probed, prodded, tested and advised by a plethora of professionals. As I have mentioned in various parts of this book, the experiences and the answers were not always what I wanted or expected, and sometimes the experiences were downright unpleasant. In truth, though, I was in the centre of a maelstrom, the focus being always on me and the target being always to get me better. Whether you like it or not, if you go through that kind of intense focus for a sustained period of time, you not only become reliant on it, there is also a sad little part of you that takes great comfort and joy from it - not quite the meaning of the Christmas carol, but, if I am to be totally honest, that is how I felt. Everyone has a little of Shrek's donkey in them, 'Pick me, Pick me, Pick me'. It is all-encompassing – both the disease and the subsequent treatments, so that you cannot help but be caught up in it; the good, the bad and the downright melodramatic. Now I cannot say that anyone else will feel the same as me, even if they have similar paths in their dealings with cancer. Maybe it is because I am single and alone that the form of direction and security the NHS blanket wrapped round me meant that I clung to it like a two-year-old does to their favourite teddy bear. I am no psychologist, but maybe I enjoyed the attention; maybe I enjoyed the positive comments on how I was being so brave and stoic in my dealings with this nasty disease - mummy's brave little soldier. The simple fact is that I had been so wrapped up in an affair with the disease, the NHS and more importantly some truly amazing individuals that, almost as with the end of a relationship, I was left feeling abandoned, wanting, scared and isolated. I was now just another soul with some medical issues that needed addressing, and that separation from close cosseting to average Joe Bloggs patient was very frightening to me.

As with most things that happen to me in my life, and as I have mentioned before, I always try to just roll with the punches and accept, try to understand and sometimes embrace the changes that happen to me. I set my mind to doing the same with the latest development in my treatments. I tried to focus on the positive elements of my future by doing what I thought was best: I hit the pub! My friends Jo and Mof got married, and, after a few drinks at the reception, I suddenly realised that I could still knock back a few and drift into the ever welcoming warm arms of alcoholic-induced overconfidence. For quite a while after my last long stay in hospital at the start of April, I had sensed a drifting from certain friendships, and small things would happen that would avalanche in my brain until they became tidal waves of self-believed misfortune and hurt. I have said that I stopped updating people by text about how things had been going, as I believed in my head that things had just drifted on too long, like Big Brother: please end this depravity and spare us the humiliation! I felt that people might even think that I was deliberately exaggerating things and that every small issue was the tip of a huge iceberg in which people were slowly but surely losing their patience with me and the whole situation. The outcome was that I felt very sorry for myself. Don't they realise that I'm doing this all alone, like some weird version of Greta Garbo?

Despite dealing with the physical aspects of my treatments and the issues I had had with some NHS staff, I now had to deal with the fact that I was starting to irritate and annoy my friends, or so I believed. One thing that did annoy me though, was every time I tried to explain the latest problems I had encountered during a procedure or appointment or hospital stay, certain people would just look at me as if I were making the majority of it up. I was indeed turning into a moany old git, but I felt it was justified in some cases, but that wasn't quite reciprocated by some friends. The end result was that I started to question myself and to dislike myself for it. So I did what I knew best: I drank. I went out and visited some pubs I had not been to in quite some time and had a couple of days where I just tried to be me, the person I had been before Mr C had popped up and said 'Eh oop, lad.' A brilliant side-effect of alcohol is that it works almost as well as some of the pain medication I take, so for the hours I was out, pain was not really an issue (well, at least after the first couple and until I got home.) I caught up with some people I had not seen for a while; they were not the close friends I refer to, but there was still a niggling little voice in the back of my head trying to convince me that they would have heard from our mutual friends that I was now a moany old bugger, but, if they had, they didn't say. Quite the opposite, as I was warmly shaken by the hand and complimented on how well I was looking (a phrase I have learnt to detest, but more on that later).

I tried to have fun; tried to drink the amounts I was once famous for; tried to crack jokes and again be the funny guy in the pub. In truth, I just tried to be me again. The result was that I realised very quickly what I knew deep down (no, I had no idea about Cliff and what he kept in the shadows) I simply realised I no longer was me. I didn't accept it as permanent, but I knew I couldn't do those sorts of things any more. I realised I couldn't, after crawling home and spending four days of just drinking water, constant vomiting and pain. It was then that I saw Nicki Minaj's arse; I really had sunk that low. After I eventually crawled away from the toilet feeling like a film star (unfortunately a cross between Charlie Sheen and Lindsay Lohan), I decided that I needed to get things sorted; I needed to form a plan going forward. Again this may have been my brain reverting to the what's-the-next-stage mode, or it may have just been a requirement to start doing something, but either way, it felt like I was taking back some form of control.

The original belief had been that I had my oesophagectomy and that it might take up to six months to recover. We were now in month 7, and I still could not see an immediate return to work or indeed any sense of my old life. As I have said previously, work had been very good up until now, and I had been receiving my normal pay, so bills etc. had not been a concern. However, I was now worried that, if things continued to drag on, this might not continue to be the case, and if my income was to disappear I was very aware that I couldn't go on *I'm a Celebrity* to revitalise my career. My biggest worry was that, as my flat was privately rented, I would not be able to keep it, as the benefits I would receive would not cover the rent.

The fact that I was sometimes stuck in the flat had always been an issue and a worry for me, and the medical staff were aware of the problem. Several times nurses had visited me, and, like a marathon runner who's just crossed the finish line and is being approached by an eager interviewer, their eyes pleaded, 'Give me five minutes please.' I believe that it was for that reason, and the fact I lived alone, that a lot of my hospital stays were sometimes a little longer than if I had been living with someone and in more appropriate surroundings. I had considered getting myself on the council housing-list a few times previously during my illness, but I didn't see how I would be able to get somewhere, despite being diagnosed with cancer, as even that would not have given me enough points to be in a reasonable position to get myself somewhere. What do points mean? Prizes! Now, however, I really did have some very worrying mobility and health-issues, so I took the plunge and filled out the application-form. My hope was just to get somewhere that didn't have stairs, with the added benefit of my being able to keep it financially if the worst happened and I could no longer count on a salary from my work.

Occasionally something happens that kicks your life down a different path, like winning the lottery or having a lobotomy or getting a contract to talk vapidly on *The Only Way is Essex*. As I have said a few times, I tend to roll with these things and sometimes it can cause regret, but sometimes it is the right nudge at the right time that really multiplies into a possible life-changing series of events. I really do believe that is very true. As I said, I applied to the council, and things were physically pretty poo, but emotionally I wasn't too bad. I was again looking forward and focusing on the next thing. As part of my application to the council, I obviously included the medical issues, and they needed contact details for verification, so I gave them details for Dr Waters, Mr Gossage and Sue. Not wanting it to be a surprise for them (like a Dyson on Christmas Day), I rang Sue to let her know and hoped that she didn't mind. Quite the opposite, Sue was really happy I was making plans and trying to get my obviously inappropriate accommodation needs resolved. Sue then said that there was a form that the oncology department social worker (I was about as aware a social worker existed as I am on the location of the mythical G-spot) could fill in for me to help improve my chances. Honest, ladies, I lie like a PPI salesperson - about the H-spot, not the form. The next day I received a blank form from the social worker, Kerry, with a note asking me to sign and date it and she would complete it and pass any other relevant information to the council on my behalf. I duly did this and awaited the outcome. The unfortunate thing was that after that I couldn't really see anything else I could do to move my life forward.

My medical problems were what they were, and the relevant parties were looking into things for me, but some of it was just the process of healing. I couldn't make any plans to return to work, as I just wasn't ready, and, like an arthritic Resident of Barbados, I was stuck in limbo! It was at this point I started to fall into the previously mentioned trough of depression. Nothing huge or crippling, but enough to make me feel as in control as Justin Bieber and as emotional as Gwyneth Paltrow at an awards' ceremony: when trains become sentient, you can emotionally uncouple Gwen. As time drifted, I slowly began to wallow in self-pity. I struggled physically to do even the basics, such as keeping on top of the housework. I had little or no motivation to do anything. At the start of my recovery I had decided to write this book, and I had bought a small electric piano to relearn, as dad had tried teaching me when I was young, and that was about as successful as the Sinclair C5. Both of these things waned, and I found myself staring at the TV without really watching and having long soaks in the bath just to break up the day. Visitors were few on the ground, either because I had put them off by being Mr Grumpy or because they simply had busy lives of their own. Either way I was quite alone. I took comfort in the routine I had now created of TV, bath, pain medication and bed. The pain had really started to become an issue now, and I had got to the point where I was taking a considerable amount of morphine. The worrying thing was, it was getting to the point that I wasn't quite sure I needed to take the amounts I was taking. I needed to know that an hour after taking it I could lie in bed, with some crap old film, and drift into oblivion where there was no pain and I didn't have to worry or stress about the future: a bit like a normal day for some Chelsea-ites.

This had been going on for a few weeks when, out of the blue, I received a call from Sue, my specialist nurse. At first I was panicky, thinking that some initial test was incorrect, or worse she was going to make them take away my pain-relief: after all, like Rihanna, I was no longer under her umbrella. It turned out that Sue just wanted to have a chat and see how things were. This is what I mean by this lady being special, along with many others in the NHS. We did what they do at Prime Minister's Question Time and danced round the issues for a bit, but then I just broke down and sobbed like a small child that truly believes the only present he has got for Christmas is the Jaggedy Arse Balaclava knitted by his great aunt Nora (thank you for that, Mr Connolly!). I couldn't help myself; Sue has such a caring nature that comes across when you talk to her that you instantly lower your defences. I'm serious: the UN should hire her; there would be fewer boundaries than an open marriage. What also stunned me, apart from the fact I didn't see any reason she should be ringing me, was that she was also one of the people that I thought had turned away from me through my moaning about past events. Whether or not I had indeed cheesed her off, I don't think I shall ever know, but, as far as Sue was concerned, I was still in need of help, and she and her department would give it for as long as I needed it. It was when she said this that I fell to pieces more quickly than

Humpty Dumpty in the incident of the high building and the ex-girlfriend. We talked for a while, and, I managed to get some sentences out between the huge sobs and the waterfall of mucous. How attractive, I hear you say! Sue had more patience than a hypochondriac's GP; she listened and was calm and helpful. The upshot was that she really thought that I needed to talk to someone professional about all this, and, after my giving her the I-don't-do-touchy-feely rubbish defence for a while, a little part of my brain began screaming, 'You need help; take it!' So I relented.

It was arranged that the QEQM oncology counsellor would give me a call and arrange something. I waited nervously for the call from this counsellor, bearing in mind my previous encounter, but I calmed myself with the thought that at least this time I wouldn't be receiving the call at work. Shortly afterwards I was called by a lady called Maureen Potter (no relation to the wheelchair-bound northern club proprietor). Maureen seemed very nice and suggested we book an appointment, with no agenda, so I could just see whether it was something that I might find useful. A week or so later I went to meet Maureen at Canterbury Hospital in a little room just behind the chemotherapy ward. I felt strange walking to the appointment through this ward, seeing people going through what I had twice previously. (No, they weren't all trying to down a bottle of Bacardi.) I felt slightly like an intruder being in the midst of these souls having their own personal cocktail of poisons drip into them like some weird episode of *ER*. I shouldn't be there when I was now cancer-free. A bit like a bloke in his twenties who gets on the wrong boat and ends up playing bingo for two weeks with the rest of the Saga Rose; shocking thing is, he's now married to Vera, 68, from Scunthorpe.

I met Maureen, and she made me feel relaxed and at ease. Maureen had a good way of coming across as interested but not overbearing. I had no idea what to expect from these meetings, but I was slightly disappointed that there was no couch and she didn't wear spectacles sitting just at the end of her nose. I did, however, see a box of tissues on the table next to me, and immediately a one-liner Frankie Boyle would have been proud of was on my lips, but I managed to stop myself from casting the words into the room. Quite simply Maureen gently probed me on how I was medically and what I had been doing about things generally, and, despite my worst fears, it just turned into my rambling on about all and sundry for the next while; some of which didn't even seem relevant. Before I knew it, like a man whose pools had come up, with a packet of three and a couple of Viagra in his bloodstream, my hour was up. We agreed a date for my next appointment the following week, and I went outside to wait for my transport home and mulled over what had just happened. The thing about me (and lots of my friends with ears as red as the Russian flag will testify to it) is that, when I haven't seen anyone for a while, as was now the case, I could quite easily outtalk Jeremy Paxman on speed. That's what Maureen had just done. There were no deep probing questions, no let's-get-in-touch-with-your-inner-child-type rubbish; she just let me waffle and vent my spleen slightly.

I continued seeing Maureen weekly for some time, and, yes, as the sessions developed, we touched on issues that were directly affecting me, but generally it didn't feel as if I were being counselled. It felt as if I had a new friend in my corner who not only empathised with what I was going through but also helped me make sense of the whys and wherefores - even if they were at my suggestion. Obviously, like a blind man in a maze, I was nudged in the right direction every now and then, but it just helped me to get a better perspective on things. And no, the tissues never got used. I didn't cry once!

During this period I had also received a couple of calls from Sue, just to see how I was, and Kerry the social worker had called just to check on me as well. So there I was, still with ongoing physical problems and still struggling to cope with the fallout of those issues but feeling better knowing I had three people in my corner courtesy of QEQM Hospital Oncology Department, Margate: Sue, Maureen and Kerry. As time went by, I kept looking on the council website every fortnight to bid on any eligible properties I could, but it seemed that they were all unsuitable for me because of the medical needs I had, or there was always someone in front of me that had been waiting longer. I couldn't understand why someone would be in the same band as me for medical reasons and that they could have been waiting for so long. It was only later, when I eventually got myself a place, that I discovered several people had viewed it prior to me and rejected it. It was then that I realised why there are some people that are on the list for such a long time. They are obviously waiting for that top-floor room to become available at Buckingham Palace. That something that is decent and meets the criteria set in their application is open to them is not quite good enough. They are like some idiots on dating sites: out of touch with reality and always positive there is something better. As the Rolling Stones so eloquently put it: People, you can't always get what you want; you get what you need.

At this time, which I shall refer to as my 'blue period' - and not because I now felt physically strong enough for some 'one love' - I had slipped into an unhealthy routine, as mentioned before. I would get up; confirm I had no medical appointments; wallow around in self-pity for a while; stare at the TV like Bob Geldof's character in a Pink Floyd video; then shuffle off and dose up when the pain got too much; go to bed and lie in wait of that relief and ability to drift like a Cuban refugee that the said pills gave me. On good days I would try and take a slow walk into town to get some essentials, or maybe just to get some human contact, but this invariably brought the pain on more quickly than a refund demanded at a Justin Bieber concert. The worst thing about this period was that the smallest thing could make me fall into the trough of depression, and, once there, I had little motivation to climb out.

I kept seeing Maureen, and that definitely helped. Then one day she suggested I apply for a benefit I might be able to get, called PIP (Personal Independence Payment). Maureen filled in the relevant form based on my situation and sent it off. This lifted my spirits, as it could mean I would be given help to get around. A mobility scooter was mentioned, but quite frankly I would have rather been cast as a love interest on an episode of *Love Island* where the stars where Louis Walsh, Jedward and Jordan than be seen driving around in one of those things. What I really hoped for was the ability to just jump in a cab when I had been out and just couldn't manage the walk home. I must point out here, and it seemed silly when it was first mentioned to me, but always be aware that, if you go walking and are not in your physical prime, every journey has a return leg. Many times I would bimble down to the seafront and start to wane, before realising that, like ET, both physically and mentally, I had to get home! The upshot of this application was I now had two positives to focus on, the move and the PIP. So, like a confused adolescent dolphin, I was now trying to get some porpoise.

It was the middle of September that I was delivered a bit of a knock that I struggled to deal with. As mentioned, my work had been fantastic so far and I was happy because there was an insurance policy in place that was covering my wages, however like Sarah Palin debating global warming, I was very wrong. My department at work had lost a couple of members of staff in my absence, and the personnel had been reshuffled, but they were having problems when Steve, who ran things in my absence, left for a career change. They were struggling to find a replacement so I received a call one Monday afternoon out of the blue. It was about half 4 and I had just allowed the morphine to replace my pain with blurry thoughts of new flats and dancing girls when said call came through. It was from my manager and he was with the HR manager from head office and I was on speakerphone so straight away, I knew something was amiss. The office structure was that I ran my department and Martin, who I mentioned having a heart operation at St Thomas,' ran the other, but as the company had been having problems recruiting, they had decided to restructure things. There would now be one overall supervisor and two 'senior' clerks. I was informed that I would automatically be given the roll of 'senior' clerk but asked if I would like to apply for the roll of overall supervisor, the admin side of the job I already did but there would be no more money. Whilst trying to deal with this set of information, I suddenly had the strangest feeling that I was being ambushed. I tried to explain that I was hoping to be back soon but I really couldn't say when and I didn't feel able at that time to give a straightforward yes or no, so they took that as being able to rule me out. I was just trying to catch up with that conversation when Cherrie the HR lady also dropped the bombshell that the insurance company hadn't been paying all my salary. They had, in fact, only been paying half and the company had been topping it up since my operation in January, and unfortunately they would no longer be doing this as from my next pay day, so therefore my gross salary would only be the half, which was what the insurance company was paying. After exchanging pleasantries, and them 'wishing me well' I hung up and tried to figure out what just happened.

I know that I have been very lucky with work doing what they had up to then, and I am very aware that lots of other companies would have stuck to the rules; I know this to be the case as when I emailed work about gross amounts etc after this conversation, it was pointed out very clearly to me what they could have done regarding my pay in the previous months since my oesophagectomy. I then found out that I was owed some holiday pay which I could have split over the three remaining paydays of the year, so at least I didn't have to panic until the years end, or so I thought. I also found out that the latest property I had bid on was quite popular and there were a few people in front of me, so unable to stop myself, I went from riding the waves, to being engulfed by them very quickly. Now I haven't gone into details about the work thing or the house thing to make you say poor me. I was very lucky that work had supported me so long and I was also very lucky that the QEQM team had helped me with the housing and the mobility application. To be truthful I wasn't in a great position, but I certainly wasn't destitute. The reason I mention this is that, on top of my general sense of loss and isolation, these things combined to plunge me headlong into a state of despair that I had never experienced before and hope never to again. Usually at the end of that last sentence I would have added a pun to lighten the mood but to be honest, like Borat at a UN conference, it just wasn't appropriate; bugger, just done one. Hello, darkness my old friend, the song, not Jeremy Clarkson welcoming the band on a fast lap test. As I have mentioned before, most people have the ability to see over the edge of the trough of depression and eventually claw their way out. Others simply can't and don't; this is where I now found myself. The general low state of my existence; the news from work; the fact that I believed I wasn't going to get the home I hoped for and the general absence of human contact had taken me very quickly to a place so low I expected to see a sign saying, 'Welcome to Katie Hopkins' Home.' In all seriousness though, it is very surprising how lots of little things can soon become one huge thing, and your ability to function, or indeed want to function, can disappear quicker than an investment maintained by Lehman Brothers. Suicide is a word that I never thought for one second would be included in this book. After all, I had just spent 14 months, accepting, planning and dealing with this awful disease to be able to regain the life I had; so why on earth, after all that, would I even contemplate that awful word? The simple fact is that I did. For those of you who don't follow plots very well; I didn't follow it through, that's why you're reading this. The fact is I simply couldn't cope any more, but unfortunately I also knew I couldn't end my life. Not because so many people had worked so hard to save it already; not because of the people who would be left behind to pick up the pieces, but quite simply, I couldn't because of my relationship with God. I was terrified of going to hell based on all the stupid things I thought I had already done in my life; I definitely didn't want to get an admittance ticket based on ending the greatest thing I had been given- life itself. The problem was that rather than lift me, this thought seemed to make the situation even bleaker. The only way out I could see was not open to me. I feel I must say here that I know people who have made the decision to take their own lives; my thoughts are purely my thoughts based on the faith I have, conflicting with other theories I have, but in essence my thoughts alone. I don't know if what I believe is fact, and until the day I do die I will never know. I just have strong feelings of faith that I allow to guide me. My faith isn't ruled by dogma, or the 'rantings' that some have drilled into them at an early age. My beliefs are based on my years of trying to understand my faith and to understand myself. The fact is I felt a little like Job; for those unfamiliar, he was the guy whose loyalty God and the Devil decided to test by doing some pretty awful things to him; sort of like a Bush tucker trial but on a global scale. Again, as if to emphasise the point of religion and dogma, I don't believe that any God I could have a relationship with could be as callous as to put one of his most loved children through such ordeals just to say, 'I told you so,' to the Devil; yet it is in the Bible. I also struggle to love a God that can ignore such pain and suffering that endures every day on this planet. I struggle to make science and what we have learnt harmonise with religion. The only thing that appeases my brain is faith. I believe that there are reasons for things happening; no matter how horrendous. I believe that when I die it may all become clear to me; if, that is, I manage to get my name on the entry list. The theory of unification is what Einstein died trying to prove, (and like a Sun journalist with a hacked phone basis of knowledge) don't quote me on this, it is a way of understanding how the very small things around us, such as in Quantum Mechanics, and the very big things such as Gravity and electromagnetism work together. We know they do as the universe exists, but no one has yet proven it; the closest physicists have come I believe is String Theory. The fact is, like unification, things exist and happen and just because we cannot identify and pinpoint exactly why, doesn't mean that they don't. I do not compare myself to someone worthy of God's personal attention, although my faith tells me otherwise, but that is where I was- between the proverbial rock and a hard place.

Now please don't panic people! Like the man with a one inch willy, that's about as deep as I go. So I did the only thing I felt I could, I reached out to the people who had been so supportive of me during that period, Sue, Kerry and Maureen. I wrote emails as it was late in the day and I don't think I could talk to them anyway. Also I found writing things down was extremely cathartic, and looking back at the emails, it now makes me realise how small the individual problems were, but as I said, at the time they were mountains. I didn't expect replies straight away due to the hour and the day, but as soon as I had unburdened myself, so to speak, I felt a lot better. I was still lower than the latest Voice winner's debut single, but I had released some of my burden and therefore my tension.

The following Monday I tentatively waited for the fallout from my emails, but like most X Factor finals, there was no great pinnacle. I think that it was due to the context of things, and the fact I had a previously booked doctor's appointment that Monday morning, that when I received a reply from Kerry, who was obviously concerned, she had contacted my GP and thought that I would be best talking things through with him. Now my GP was a nice enough chap, and thanks to him I had received an early diagnosis of my cancer, but I wasn't sure that I could confide all in him. Despite the fact I didn't want to admit things out loud, I had always found talking to women a lot easier than to men; probably some cave-man instinct, but that was me. Anyway I went to see him, and he tentatively broached the subject in a very gentle way. I found myself being quite honest with him, and apart from the lump the size of a melon in my throat, I did feel better. He prescribed me some anti-depressants; a mild one that also had the benefit of being a sedative so I might get some better sleep; and we parted company with me seeing a glimmer of silver on the clouds hovering over Dover Harbour. The truth is (and it's an old cliché) there is always a light at the end of every tunnel. That is unless the tunnel in question is Mr Slave and the object travelling through said tunnel is Lemmiwinks; sorry, had to get at least one South Park based pun in there. I had felt a little disappointed in the reaction from my three favourite NHS staff at that time, but what I didn't know was the work these three wonderful people had been doing on my behalf, not only since they had first met me but also subsequent to my awful weekend and the emails I had then sent. The upshot was that Sue called me in her extremely gentle and caring way and we had a long chat; well she chatted and I blubbed like Paris Hilton when she realised her latest self-released 'home movie' had not gone viral. Also Maureen and Kerry had gone into overdrive chasing up my PIP application.

The light (or I should say incandescence) that hit me over the next few weeks was as positive to me as all the negatives combined. Firstly, I was just leaving hospital after a meeting with Maureen and I received a call from the council asking me if I was still interested in the property I had applied for a few weeks previously. I said that I was, and the very next day I went to view it. It was perfect; a one bedroom bungalow in a lovely village about 5 miles out of Dover. The only apprehension I had was that I had to take the tenancy a week later so I might lose the deposit on my previous flat, and also getting about would be a little difficult due to its location. However, as I said about the people ahead of me on the list, I wasn't going to hope for perfect; I was going to take what I needed. The fact that it was perfect was just the icing on the cake; like meeting a gorgeous girl who likes you and then realising she has a trust fund. I had previously warned my existing landlord that I was looking for alternative accommodation for obvious reasons a few months prior, so after some 'let's be reasonable' conversations, I did get my deposit back and they got 10 days money already paid as compensation. Kerry advised me to speak to a subsidiary branch of Macmillan to see if they could assist with the move. At the time I was at St Thomas' in London having the procedure and chat with Mr Gossage, and the lovely team of three that cover Macmillan in my area went into overdrive and arranged for a local company to move me, and they said that they were going to cover the initial cost if I could reimburse them half later on, which I was more than happy to do. When I was signing all the paperwork to take possession of the new house, the lady doing this advised me that I may even get some help with things from SSAFA (Soldiers, Sailors and Air Force Association) as I had served some years in the RAF. I thought this highly unlikely as it was 30 odd years previously and I had only served 5 and half years. I did, however, make a request to them and was very surprised that after some checks they paid for my carpets, a new washing machine, gave me an Argos voucher to get other things I needed for the new place and they paid Macmillan back the full cost of my move. So thank you SSAFA and the RAF Benevolent Fund. I must point out that I did feel uncomfortable about taking them up on this very kind offer initially, as I didn't feel that my needs quite matched someone returning from abroad with some awful life-changing injury. However, David, the nice chap who arranged everything, pointed out that what I may receive would not in any way take from someone who needed it more, so that appeased my conscious a lot. Just when I didn't think I could get any more sets of 6 lottery numbers, I had an email from Kerry, my social worker, informing me that I had indeed qualified for the PIP allowance and I would receive the letter shortly. Seems she had been chasing it on my behalf and had cut down my wait time quite considerably. So, there I was mid-October, a month after wasteland weekend, and I had a beautiful new home; the anti-depressants were indeed helping me sleep and taking the edge from things and I now had the ability to look at mobility.

I hope that I haven't gone into too detailed a diatribe of personal self-pity and 'woe is me' in this section because that really is not the intention. I don't say things to seem a victim and I don't want to come across as a petulant child who stamps his feet when things don't go his way. The simple fact is that all of these things happened to me in a relatively short period post my all clear. I want to impress on you that this point of your dealings with Cancer could possibly be as internally traumatic; I use this phrase because on the outside looking in, things may not have appeared so bad, but from where I was looking out, they were awful.

I had some fantastic support from the fantastic three at QEQM; I did have friends who called and supported me at very low points - thank you, Kris, Dave, Graham, Chris, Mof and of course Ange. I have an amazing set of cousins, who have always tried to be there and of course our kid Shirley and Dom. The fact is that no one did anything wrong, no one was better at being a friend than anyone else. Some just coped better and knew when to make the calls that mattered.

I have thought long and hard about exactly how I got out of the trough I was in this time, for myself as a self-help tool if ever it were to happen again, but also to give you pointers if it should ever happen to you. All I can do is say this. I got out for many reasons, I believe. I realised that I was indeed in a trough, so I sought help. Thanks to the Fabulous Three (no, not what's left of Take That) at the QEQM, I had somewhere to turn to. However, the most fortunate thing that happened is that my personal situation started to turn: I was having positive things happen to me rather than negatives. So, like some psychological stabilisers, I began to get myself back on track. Quite how the medication works I don't really know, but it definitely seemed to take the edge off things. Importantly, though, in my limited knowledge of such things, I don't believe my depression was linked to a serious physical chemical imbalance to which many people who suffer from long term depression are usually subject. I believe that a combination of all these factors gave me the proverbial ladder to climb out. I was certainly in a better place, but I was also very aware that like Tiger's colonoscopy, I wasn't out of the woods just yet. The only suggestion I can give - and as I keep repeating, this is all based on my experience and limited knowledge – is, that if you have the chance to establish a close and supportive relationship with someone you can trust in the NHS who has the time to give you, nurture it. Do not be afraid to ask for help, any kind, from professionals to friends to family. Know what is normal for you. so that you can keep an eye out for the abnormal. Most of all, remember that things can turn around more quickly than a homophobe realising he's just joined a Gay Pride conga-line. I have gone into hospital feeling physically very poorly, and, with the right treatment and care, twenty-four hours later I was fine. I went into my own personal trough of depression over a slower period, but again, with the right treatment and care, I got out much more quickly than I believed possible. Just make sure you always keep yourself in a position to be able to get that right treatment and care if you should ever need it.

I came out of that darkness like Meatloaf's big break: no, not with 147 at snooker, but like a bat out of hell. It was only later, towards the end of the year, that I was talking to Maureen and was yet again extolling her, Sue and Kerry that I had made Dr Waters personally aware (though I'm sure he already was) that he had three of the most patient, caring and professional people working in his team that he could wish for. It was then that Maureen explained why they had put in so much effort to get me into the new home and get the transport allowance sorted. It was quite simple: I had experienced some post-op complications that were not expected. My expected recovery-plan had deviated more than Madonna's career. I had been going through some personal problems that were not expected. Lots of things had happened that were beyond my control, and, more importantly, it had all happened at a time when I was most vulnerable,- with the support mechanisms' all having being removed after my all-clear. Maureen, Sue and Kerry all knew that, if I had a better foundation, I could leave my home without fear of getting back in. I was as mobile physically as I could be, and I could get to the hospital, doctors and other appointments without having to wait around in pain for several hours before and after for transport. They knew that, if that was in place, I could cope with the rest. Like a parent with ear-muffs at a 1D concert; I would survive. This was proved to me many times in the following few months.

On 28 October I presented myself to St Thomas' to have the exploratory operation on my rib. It was done by Professor Mason, and I woke to be told that they had looked at me, had scraped away an area and put some pins in with the intention of stopping the clicking. They told me this whilst I had the biggest grin on my face, bigger than Larry Luckafella after collecting his sixth lottery win in his brand new Rolls with the nubile twenty-three-year-old Mrs Luckafella sitting next to him. The reason for my grin was not that I had met two of the loveliest nurses you could hope for when I woke in the recovery-room. The place was packed, and I had told them not to worry about me, as I could see they were busy, as it appeared that Mr Drugs Overdose from my main operation had told a lot of his friends, and they had all turned up on that day. This seemed to have the opposite effect on these two lovely nurses, and they both proceeded to fuss over me. Let me tell you that having your arm rubbed whilst being administered as much morphine as you need whilst being told what a lovely chap you are is about as close to heaven as I have ever managed to get!

The fact that everywhere was so busy meant I had to stay in the recovery-ward a lot longer than usual: bummer! Anyway, as I say, the reason for my grin was that as soon as the morphine had started to wear off and I was back at levels that a human being can tolerate, I suddenly went to move in my bed and realised: no clicking! Now I cannot stress enough how demoralising and debilitating the clicking had been. To have it disappear so swiftly was like being able to flick the off-switch on an episode of *Strictly*: heaven. There was still the pain, but at that stage I was unsure whether it was residual from the operation or whether it was permanent. I met Mr Gossage at the start of December, and I remember sitting in the waiting area of St Thomas' outpatient department waiting to go in and see him, when - click! The fact is I convinced myself that this must be psychosomatic. I must be imagining it, until - click again!

I had my meeting with Mr Gossage and, for the reasons mentioned, I decided against telling him it had just clicked. He advised me that it could take up to six months to heal fully and that because of the amount of pain-relief that they had used on the site during the operation it might still be too early to know whether the experienced pain was indeed going to subside. We arranged to meet again just after my next oncology appointment in March, and I thanked him again, whilst feeling relieved that St Thomas' really didn't have a uterus transplant department, because I was enjoying being a lot lighter. I then had some bloods taken and saw another specialist nurse on the Upper GI unit called Julie, who was extremely nice and removed the remains of a small internal stitch that had done a Kavanagh and 'come out.' I tentatively mentioned to her about the click I thought I had felt whilst waiting, and she advised me to monitor it and give her a ring if I became worried.

A few days later, the clicking had indeed returned with a vengeance. I must be honest and say that in frequency it was not so bad as it had been previously and that it appeared to be happening a few inches further round to my side, but it was indeed like Mr Schwarzenegger: back. I decided to seek some advice from Julie at St Thomas', and she said I could come back up to see Mr Gossage straightaway if it would help, but in truth there wasn't much that could be done, as I had enough pain-relief on prescription. I told Julie that I had agreed to see Mr Gossage again in three months and mentioned that he had stated it could take up to six months to repair fully. I added that it was probably best I stick to that, and she agreed but said I should contact her if things deteriorated. The fact is that the clicking has deteriorated and the pain is again an issue. I waited for the trough of depression to slide into my home like a door-to-door salesman who spots an open door and takes it as a personal invite for him to pitch. The thing is, it didn't come. I bought a new kitchen and some loft-insulation, but the trough never reappeared. Maureen was right: the foundation they had put in place kept me afloat long enough to get a sense of reality and not to sink.

Chapter Twelve
Personal Advice

Do as I say, not as I do! The fact is, I am definitely one of those people who are very good at handing out advice but not very good at taking it, from myself or anyone else. I am quite a headstrong person, and whether it is for that reason or because I have lived alone for so long I cannot say. All I know is that I am initially about as likely to act on advice as Dave Grohl is to extol a Westlife album. I guess the simplest way to look at things is by considering what motivated me to write this book in the first place. When I first thought about writing, it was for two reasons. Firstly, I have quite a strange sense of humour (call it a coping mechanism), and, after getting over the initial impact of being diagnosed, I started remembering it in that Monty Pythonesque way that I described in the first chapter. Humour was my armour, so why can't it be someone else's? Secondly, I really do believe that, by being honest, sometimes brutally so like Jimmy Carr's tax-accountant, and by giving as true an account of my dealings with this disease as possible, I may in some small way inform, comfort and hopefully give a better sense of perspective to as many people as possible who are facing their own version of cancer. As I say many times throughout this book, I am not a writer or a medical professional, but I have a grasp of the way things have happened and the reasons behind them. I am just another soul who has had his life altered by this illness, but I want to feel as if it didn't completely change me, and, by writing about it, I am almost taking back a form of control over it.

You will hear many things in the course of your dealings with this disease, from friends, family and medical professionals. I shall mention a few that were relevant to me. One of them has been: 'You're so brave.' I certainly am not. I'm about as brave as Colonel Gaddafi when he said his next palace was 'in the pipeline'. Bravery is someone who fights for human rights and is the sole voice of reason in a crowd of hatred and nurtured intolerance, like Malala Yousafzai or Rosa Parks. Bravery is someone who defends others at personal cost, someone who battles their own personal demons day by day but never feels bitter or self-piteous. Bravery is the inner strength to know when something is not right and to try to do something about it. Bravery is a truly caring professional in the NHS who keeps giving a part of themselves every shift, every appointment, to ensure we have the best lives we can. I don't believe I am those things. I wish I were, but the truth is, I am just a person who got caught in a freak wave and clung like buggery to anything that floated There were times when I have been, and you will need to be, stoic. This, however, is not bravery: it is just the right thing to do to protect yourself, or more importantly, to protect the ones you care about.

Another one is: 'You look really good.' This particular comment has probably annoyed me more than any other during the last year or so. I know that it is said either with the best of intentions - as Chris Rea said, there's that road to hell again - or in genuine thoughtfulness, but the truth in my case is that it was almost a vindication that I was indeed a wimp. The fact is that on many occasions when it was said to me I was feeling about as 'good' as Britney Spears having a short back and sides. The problem I had with it was that it played on my emotional vulnerability: if they said I was looking good, I must be, therefore perhaps I am indeed being soft and things aren't so bad as I think they are - when in truth I was feeling awful. I believe that a lot of these comments were prompted by my weight-loss: approximately equal to a small dog or one of Mr Creosote's bowel movements (Monty Python again, people), and as a consequence I had bought some new clothes that fitted me, so I probably did look a lot better than some had remembered me.

There were, however, some that genuinely meant it, these being people that had been close to me over the months and really did see a marked difference compared with times when I had resembled the 'last chicken in Sainsbury's' (I thank you again, Mr Connolly). The fact is that no-one said it in any way other than to make me feel better, but the truth is that a lot of the time I felt like the European Parliament: looking good on the outside but a messed-up bag of conflicting, directionless confusion on the inside. The way I dealt with it was to smile politely, thank them but add that it's not such a rosy picture from my side of the window. It really depends on who you are talking to, as hurting someone's feelings when you may need them later is never a good idea. (Take note, Katie Hopkins: you may end up having an operation performed by a surgeon who is overweight, was once on the dole and who was educated in a comprehensive school on a council estate just outside Rotherham!)

The worst of all, however, was: 'No, Mr Bond, I expect you to die!' Oh, hang on, that wasn't said: it was in that dream I had about Pussy Galore! The thing is that many times people will say things to you that slide on some weird comfort scale from slightly uncomfortable to downright cringe-worthy.

You have to take things in context. As I have said before, people singular are quite extraordinary and kind-hearted. If, however, you don't think you will cause offence, be honest. Don't bite the hand that feeds you, but a gentle nibble could make a difference. One thing I shall suggest, though, regards your dealings with the medical professionals. Don't be afraid to question things. If someone tells you something about your plan or treatments and you are unsure or disagree, say something. You don't have to be rude or impolite (take note, Mr Paxman), but this is about you and your life. They will not be annoyed if you ask a genuine question or need clarification. Since it is important that you understand what is happening to you so that you can deal with it, speak up when you have the opportunity and ensure you are as aware of things as you can be, like a someone pretending to be blind at a naturist camp. Before appointments with doctors, nurses etc, write down the questions you need answering and take them with you to the appointments. There's nothing more frustrating (other than not having the remote to hand during a Cameron party broadcast) than getting home afterwards and thinking, bugger, I wish I'd asked about that! What I think you need to be aware of is that nothing said to you is meant to do anything other than help you. As I have said before, I sometimes felt, whether rightly or wrongly, that friends could have done more; but the fact is they did the best they could.

Friendship is a precious and important part of anyone's life, and, like any relationship, it requires work. That you are now a constant reminder of every human being's basic fear – cancer or similar - adds a new dynamic to the relationship. You will be pleased, happy and disappointed with friends throughout your life; this is normal. So why should you not have these same emotions with friendships just because you're ill? I was particularly upset because over my treatments and recovery I had two birthdays. The first was before I knew the tumour was operable, and the second was after I had my all-clear but was in a pretty dark place. On the first birthday I was recovering from my laparoscopy and was a bit sore, but I still thought I should have a wave of people coming round or trying to get me out to celebrate, but, like an extremist meeting Mr Tolerance and getting on like a house on fire, it just didn't happen. My second birthday (no, not the one where I still wore nappies and acted like Nikki Grahame from Big Brother) was better, as friends took me to a local jam night and I was having quite a good day health-wise, so had a few drinks, sang a couple of songs and had a great time; but the friends I most expected to be knocking on my door, didn't. Again, they let my birthday drift by. The fact is that the friends I had expected, or hoped, would make the effort didn't, but, when I thought about things, they hadn't in previous years, so why now just because I have cancer? As I say, relationships require work and effort from both sides; just because you're ill doesn't change that, much as you may want it to.

One thing I have struggled to cope with, and still worry about, is the 'irrational' fear of the cancer's returning. I put the word irrational in inverted commas because it really is not that irrational. You have looked the devil in the eye and told him to shove it, so quite naturally, like an Aussie trying to lose a razor-bladed boomerang, you would be terrified of its returning with a vengeance. The main issue with me was that some of the symptoms that led to my needing a dilatation (widening of the pipes: think new lane on the M25) reminded me of symptoms I experienced prior to my original diagnosis: pain in the chest, eating issues etc. No matter how many times a specialist explains it to you, it is quite natural to worry. I write this on the eve of my next dilatation at St Thomas' Hospital, and even now, with all the facts, there is still a small part of my brain that thinks they are going to find a new growth, and this time it will be 'game over'. The only advice I can offer on this is to maintain that contact between you and one of the specialists who dealt with you. I don't mean to the extent you ring them every time you experience a twinge, like some terrified hypochondriac or Michael Owen during his Man Utd period, as we like to call him. Keeping the communication-lines open between you and someone in the NHS who knows what you have dealt with, or are indeed continuing to deal with, will give you the peace of mind and assurance that you may need from time to time. Trust me, the good ones will not mind; it's what they are there for.

Dependent on the type of cancer and subsequent treatment you have, you may find yourself in a situation similar to mine. No, I don't mean craving human contact but settling for a cat, but you may have had some serious alteration to your bodywork, like some extreme version of *Pimp My Ride*. These physical changes can be quite a shock to deal with. In my case, they took part of my stomach that showed signs of cancer cells (sounds like some extreme prison on Guantanamo Bay), made a small pouch for food and used the rest to make me a new oesophagus. The result is that I obviously cannot eat as much as I should like. Now this is great for keeping the weight down, but getting the balance and eating the right things is an act that I am still trying to get to grips with. I used to love going out for meals, but now it scares me. As I haven't quite got to grips with it yet, if I have a full plate in front of me I will eat till I feel full, but instead of stopping there, part of me still feels hungry or is simply enjoying the taste of whatever it is, and I think I'll just have a little bit more - until the plate is finished, and I end up doing an impression of Harry Styles minus the freeway. At home this is very controllable, as I just use side-plates now for my meals. That said, it's amazing how much you can squeeze on to a side plate (a bit like Kim Kardashian, I imagine, trying on medium-sized knickers). If you do have similar problems, then speak to your specialist: again another reason for keeping that link open, they may be able to help you. In my case I now have a small card that states my basic issues and requests the restaurant to assist me by letting me order a child's portion. This saves me the temptation a full plate gives and also avoids the embarrassment of having three-quarters of my meal returned to the kitchen and the chef thinking I am ruder than an octogenarian at a mixed-race street-party.

I don't know what the real you was like prior to getting and hopefully beating cancer, but for me I was a pepperami: a bit of an animal. I don't mean I used to stay out all night, drink from puddles and pee up trees to mark my territory. Oh, hang on, there was that stag do in '89 … I mean I used to work so that I had a social life. I went out whenever I could afford it; even many times when I couldn't; I drank far more than I should, and I scythed a bar with my rapier wit. (OK, I cracked the odd joke.) My social life revolved round my friends, my music and pubs. Now here I was with little or no inclination to go out and, even if I did, I was a shell of the person I had been. The constant fatigue, pain, eating issues and psychological problems combined to make me feel I should never be myself again. The truth is, I shan't, and that is where the physical changes can be difficult to accept, let alone deal with. I try to cope with this by telling myself that I am lucky and changes don't matter, because the fact is I am still here.

Unfortunately, whilst that does help you make sense of it, it doesn't always work. Wanting the best from life and what it has to offer is a basic human instinct. That doesn't mean financially or materialistically: the best of life means different things to different people; that's why we are so diverse and incredible. So, despite my handing my brain the I-survived-and-others-didn't card, I was also secretly wanting more but was too scared to admit it to myself or to others for fear of being labelled a Heather Mills: ungrateful and greedy. I was at a point where what I was now needed to change. That scared me at first, but the more I talked it through with Maureen my counsellor and other professionals, the more I realised that it may be a huge thing, but, if I just accept it, I can learn to accommodate it in whatever comes next for me. My physical being wasn't what defined me totally before, otherwise I'd still be a virgin, and it won't define me totally going forward. My mind and my emotions are me. The body is a tool to achieve what the true self wants. I call this the apologetic Marianas Trench philosophy. Sorry: very deep!

After all the treatments are done and all the counselling and support you may need is finished, you are back to where you were just before diagnosis: just you. The only difference is that you may now have a totally different set of aims or a new perspective on how you interact or are with things. Either way there is just you and your life, so get on with it. Enjoy it, but maybe breathe a little harder, love a little longer, be a little more true to yourself and your loved ones. Reach a little further, but most importantly be you and live. Countries don't fight for a piece of land then let it rot and go barren, so don't fight for your life and then ignore it. Live: you've earned it!

Most important for me, and I hope for you, is to thank those who have given so much help to you throughout your ordeal, both personal and professional. Yes there will be negatives but, as I have said before, you will come across some remarkable people and, if we can say thank you to someone who holds a door open for us, we can make the time to say thank you to the important people who got us through one of the darkest chapters in our lives. It doesn't have to be a grand gesture; the words 'Thank You' are often enough. If a nurse or a department has touched you, give them a card or a box of chocolates. If a specialist has made a difference, tell their superior; they don't do it for that reason, but positive feedback in any job is always appreciated. If you have a special talent that can help, offer it. I sang at the chemotherapy ward Christmas do, not for praise but because it felt as if I were giving something back: something small, but something. I gave cards and chocolates to people as a small token, but it had a big impact. I have spoken to Macmillan, SSAFA, my counsellor Maureen and Sue my specialist nurse and asked whether there was anything I could do to help. I don't particularly mean fundraising. I wanted to know whether I could perhaps be on the end of a phone for someone going through similar; just something personal to feel as if I were giving them back a small percentage of the time they had invested in me. Look back over your treatment and seek out those that deserve a thank you and give it. Give it real good.

I have been very fortunate to have had some wonderful people by my side over the past eighteen months. OK, OK, you spotted it, but I'm not changing the book-title now. There are too many to mention all; and, knowing me, I should forget someone and end up like UKIP when people realise their lack of substance: ignored. I must, however, mention a few. So, a huge thank you to: Ange, Shirley, Dom, all of my wonderful family in Glasgow, Sue Levett and

Maureen Potter. I should especially like to mention two people for the simple reason they were a great source of help to me, despite the fact they were both dealing with very serious illness themselves: so thank you and I wish you a speedy return to a healthy life as soon as possible, John Peevor and Kerry Stuart. And finally, thanks to Beau Jangles (my cat!) for allowing me no longer to be seen talking to myself and for putting up with my moods, yet still allowing me to feed you, play with you and dispose of your bodily functions.

Chapter Thirteen
My Wish List

I have many thoughts on what I should wish for, either because of what happened to me or because something didn't. These are my personal thoughts, and, if someone reads this, either as a professional or as a person, maybe they will do something that might make a difference, large or small. One thing that really annoyed me many times throughout my dealings with cancer was the huge advertising campaigns that are constantly on television for Macmillan or Cancer Research. Of course, I in no way minded the causes being brought to people's attention, the raising of awareness or the funds being raised. Maybe it's the cynic in me, but they seemed to be on constantly, and they were obviously using major expensive London advertising-agencies to enlarge their profiles. Like a petulant child, I would stamp my feet and wonder: where's my help? The truth is, it's easy to be negative.

Macmillan helped me, as I mention before, and, if Cancer Research had not been striving so hard for so many years, would my chemotherapy have been available? Would my operation have been possible? So, the wishes I mention below are meant, like the Big Bang dating Eastenders, in the genuine hope of a positive outcome.

Macmillan. The adverts on TV used to drive me insane during my treatment. Especially the one where everyone was getting cancer and falling, then bang, out of nowhere they were caught by the Macmillan nurse. Where was my nurse? Where was my support? The fact is that Macmillan helped me twice, once with train fares to London for appointments and secondly when I needed to move house. However, as far as I am aware, there are no Macmillan nurses to help with people like me in my area. The team of three lovely dedicated people that did are a subsidiary part of Macmillan. So, my first wish is that people continue to support Macmillan, but please get in touch and ask them where the money goes. Ask them how you can directly fund these smaller subsidiaries that are vital to people in times of trouble. If you receive help from them, let Macmillan know how important what they do is.

Cancer Research UK. Shortly after my all-clear, when I was like Mark Thatcher on a rally - more than a little lost - I contacted them and asked them why I hadn't had any form of request for information from them. I then received a nice reply asking me why I enquired. The thing is, I should have thought, and maybe I am wrong, that they would have some form of database that had information relating to everything to do with a cancer-patient: age, colour, lifestyle, family history, even some physical tissue samples, or at least the results from biopsies. It was the fact that I had not been asked for any of this information that had prompted me to contact them. I received a reply saying that was not the way they worked: they were approached by professionals, doctors etc. who had an idea that they wanted funding for, and a board would consider the proposal and, if accepted, that application would receive funding. That was perfectly fine but, as I pointed out to them, would a database of such information not be a great common denominator for all research? I have not received a reply to this question, and I am sure that personal data-protection is a worry, but I for one would not object to being on such a database if it were to give a basis of general information that could be collated and observed in the hope of helping with research. Would you? So my wish here is that you contact Cancer Research and ask the same question, or better still, that they look into it and see whether it is possible.

I am unsure what may happen to me now. On 19 January 2015 I returned to work on a 'phased return'. The firm are letting me work only three mornings a week, which will build as my abilities do. I wanted to return quickly, because I wanted to earn some money, but more importantly because I wanted to know my limits. I am aware that some of the physical changes are probably going to be permanent, so I need to know what I am capable of. I have found the return to work very difficult and am struggling with concentration, pain and fatigue, but that may improve, and it's early days. If it turns out I can't manage and I have to say goodbye to work for medical reasons, I'm OK with that; I shall cope. If it happens, I may go to university. I may get rich from this book! More chance of Kate Winslet realising she's made a huge mistake not finding me by taking out a full-page ad in the papers:

> Sad actress seeks folically challenged ex-ginger with great voice and wicked sense of humour for long term shag-fest. Operation-scars a positive but not mandatory.

I may finish the album some friends and I have been writing, and it may, like Alan Sugar when faced with the self-preaching ineptitude that only his show can produce in people, go ballistic. I don't know what will happen, but the truth is I wasn't very sure before I had cancer, so I'm really no better or worse off. The birds don't tweet more loudly and the trees aren't greener, but I am more aware of things in general now. I think I have more tolerance, and I definitely have a better perspective on things. I should still like to do my bucket-list: drive an Aston Martin DB9 Volante and sing with Jools Holland's band. Just thought I'd mention it again, in case it leads to offers! I still hope to meet the right woman and to re-learn the piano, but right now I am fortunate to be able to say the same as most other people: let's see what happens. Like Einstein trying to balance the books, I have plenty of time.

Personal Pledge

Part of my reason for writing this book was to be able to raise funds for cancer charities in this country. I have thought about which charity should benefit, but in the end I thought the best way to ensure it goes to even the smallest of charities was quite simple: you choose. My intention is to give 50% of all profits to cancer charities based on a pro rata scale, so please fill in the form below, and I will make sure your chosen charity gets its share. I also intend to help as many others as I can in the future, so if you wish to contact me, you can do so at the same email address as for charity nominations. I will not and cannot go into personal medical requests. I am not a doctor, but if I can help you, I shall try. I cannot assist anyone financially, but I will be very happy to help you through something I have mentioned in this book.

Charity Nomination

I…………………………………………………. nominate

……………………………………………………

Email your choice to: pquinn65@googlemail.com

Lightning Source UK Ltd.
Milton Keynes UK
UKOW02f1953230316

270760UK00001B/15/P

9 781782 284086